VIROLOGY MONOGRAPHS

DIE VIRUSFORSCHUNG IN EINZELDARSTELLUNGEN

CONTINUING / FORTFÜHRUNG VON

HANDBOOK OF VIRUS RESEARCH

HANDBUCH DER VIRUSFORSCHUNG

FOUNDED BY / BEGRÜNDET VON

R. DOERR

EDITED BY / HERAUSGEGEBEN VON

S. GARD · C. HALLAUER · K. F. MEYER

11

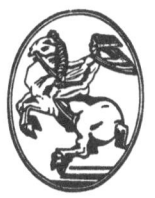

1972

SPRINGER-VERLAG

WIEN   NEW YORK

CANINE DISTEMPER VIRUS

BY

M. J. G. APPEL AND J. H. GILLESPIE

MARBURG VIRUS

BY

R. SIEGERT

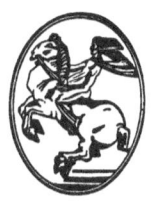

1972

SPRINGER-VERLAG

WIEN   NEW YORK

ISBN-13:978-3-7091-8304-5   e-ISBN-13:978-3-7091-8302-1
DOI: 10.1007/978-3-7091-8302-1

Canine Distemper Virus

By

M. J. G. Appel

Veterinary Virus Research Institute
Cornell University
Ithaca, New York 14850, U.S.A.

and

J. H. Gillespie

Department of Microbiology
New York State Veterinary College
Cornell University
Ithaca, New York 14850, U.S.A,

With 30 Figures

Table of Contents

I. Introduction and History

Distemper is not a very precise description of a disease entity, and the Oxford Dictionary lists a vast number of different meanings for the word "distemper": "It argues sickness and distemper in the mind as well as in the body." In connection with dogs it has been applied for centuries for "that fatal disorder proper to the canine race called par excellence, the distemper". Besides rabies, canine distemper (CD) is the only virus disease in dogs with a high mortality rate. It has a worldwide distribution and only few dogs in isolated areas remain without contact with the virus. According to some reports (KIRK, 1922; GEIGER, 1939) CD made its first appearance in Europe in Spain in 1761, introduced from either Asia or Peru. From Spain it spread to all European countries within the same century. JENNER, well known for his development of a successful smallpox vaccine, made its first accurate description in 1809.

Canine distemper is an acute or subacute contagious febrile disease with nasal and ocular discharge, gastrointestinal and respiratory signs and leukopenia. A certain proportion of affected animals develop nervous manifestations, which may occur during the acute phase of the disease or several weeks or even months later. Hyperkeratosis of foot pads is seen in some dogs. Many different species in the Order Carnivora are susceptible to CD and the mortality rate varies greatly between species.

In 1905 CARRÉ reported that canine distemper was caused by a virus. Since CARRÉ discovered the true cause of this canine disease it is known as Carré's disease. The report of CARRÉ was confirmed by LIGNIÈRES (1906). On the other hand, McGOWAN (1911), FERRY (1912), and TORREY and RAHE (1913) insisted that *Bordetella bronchiseptica (Bacillus bronchicanis)* was the primary etiological agent of canine distemper. Their filtration experiments and presumed success with a bacterin produced with *B. bronchiseptica* in the protection of dogs encouraged these investigators to believe in the bacterial etiology of this dread canine infection.

The controversy between the two divergent views continued until the classical studies of G. W. DUNKIN and Sir PATRICK LAIDLAW (1926) confirmed Carré's studies. During their distemper studies these English investigators made many notable contributions including the first use of disease-free animals reared and studied with virus infection in isolation units, an excellent description of uncomplicated distemper infection in dogs and ferrets, the production of a hyperimmune serum as a prophylaxis for dogs, and the development of an effective vaccination procedure for the immunization of dogs. The use of the ferret in canine distemper research served as a stimulus to SMITH, ANDREWES, and LAIDLAW to utilize this animal in their human influenza studies.

The excellent researches of PUNTONI (1923) went virtually unnoticed in certain countries of the world such as the United States, Great Britain, and France and still are not frequently quoted. PUNTONI showed good evidence of viral etiology when successful serial transfer in dogs resulted by the intracerebral inoculation of filtered suspensions of brain tissue. His formalin-inactivated tissue vaccine was the first one of its kind for distemper.

The contributions to canine distemper research were rather meager from 1928 until 1948. There were two exceptions: Several reports of the modification of canine distemper virus by serial passage in ferrets and the use of this attenuated virus as a vaccine for dogs appeared in the literature (WATSON, 1939; GREEN, 1939; and GREEN and SWALE, 1939); and CORDY (1942) and HURST et al. (1943) showed that canine distemper virus produced lesions in the brain of susceptible dogs.

Since 1948 many notable contributions to our knowledge of canine distemper virus and its closely related viruses — rinderpest and measles — have emerged from many laboratories in the world. These findings about canine distemper were made possible by the development of serological methods, by the propagation of the virus in hens' egg and in tissue culture, and by the development and use of brain-adapted challenge strains for the study of the disease in dogs.

The authors were fortunate to have excellent review articles (GORHAM, 1960; BINDRICH, 1954; BINDRICH, 1962) on the subject of canine distemper. The Canine Distemper Symposium (1966) of the American Veterinary Medical Association assisted greatly in presenting information about canine distemper immunity. Other common sources of information besides innumberable references in scientific journals were the short review articles by GILLESPIE (1962), and BUSSELL (1966), and the section on canine distemper by BRUNER and GILLESPIE (1966). Although we have included a large number of references no attempt was made to prepare a complete bibliography. Sufficient citations have been given so that the reader can find most of the pertinent literature.

II. Classification and Nomenclature

In the original viral classification by HOLMES (1948), canine distemper virus (CDV) was placed in the influenza group — "inducing diseases characterized principally by involvement of the respiratory tract". In the scheme proposed by the Virus Subcommittee of the International Nomenclature Committee (1963) and the Provisional Committee for Nomenclature of Viruses (ANDREWES, 1963), later adopted by the Western Hemisphere Animal Viral Characterization Committee, CDV was placed in the myxovirus group.

Various reports permitted KOPROWSKI (1958) and IMAGAWA et al. (1960) to suggest that measles virus (MV), canine distemper virus (CDV), and rinderpest virus (RV) constituted a closely-related group. COOPER (1961) suggested that the large size of measles virus and its production of inclusion bodies probably placed the measles-rinderpest-distemper (MRD) group in the herpes group as DNA viruses. Electron micrographs rendered this suggestion untenable because the three viruses were shown to have a structure quite comparable to Newcastle disease virus and other larger myxoviruses (WATERSON et al., 1961; PLOWRIGHT et al., 1962; CRUICKSHANK et al., 1962). These findings further suggested that the MRD group most likely contained an RNA rather than a DNA core. As a result, LWOFF et al. (1962) placed the MRD group among the larger myxoviruses which are RNA viruses with an envelop, helical symmetry, and a nucleocapsid of 170 mμ diameter. The Provisional Committee for Nomenclature of Viruses (ANDREWES, 1963) suggested that the Family name for this group should be *Paramyxoviridae*. WARREN et al. (1960) and GILLESPIE and KARZON (1960) found serological cross-reactions between measles and distemper in dogs. DeLay *et al.* (1965) did comparative serological studies and protection tests in various animal species with all three viruses, and their data permitted the unequivocal conclusion that the rinderpest, measles, and canine distemper viruses were closely related viruses in the family Paramyxoviridae (Table 5). MELNICK and McCOMBS (1966) called the group "medipest viruses".

III. Properties of the Virus

A. Morphology

CARRÉ (1905) was the first investigator to describe the passage of CDV through a filter that retained bacteria. LAIDLAW and DUNKIN (1926 b) first reported the unsuccessful transfer of virus through filters, but later experiments proved that CDV passed through Pasteur, Chamberland L 2, and Mandler filters. By utilizing Elford gradocol membrane the virus particle size was estimated between 70 and 105 mμ by BINDRICH and GRALHEER (1954). Applying the factor of 0.64 in the estimation of particle size in filtration experiments as recommended by BLACK (1958), PALM and BLACK (1961 b) calculated the particle size of CDV as 115 to 160 mμ.

Electron photomicrographs of CDV by CRUICKSHANK *et al.* (1962) and NORRBY *et al.* (1963) showed that their structure resembled that of the larger myxoviruses. There was a great variation in shape, but many particles were almost spherical (Fig. 1). The particles varied in diameter from 1,100 Å to 5,500 Å, although most were 1,500 Å to 3,000 Å. Intact particles showed a conspicuous outer membrane about 50—85 Å in thickness. From this outher membrane arose projections of 90—130 Å in length. In partially disrupted particles the phosphotungstate had penetrated and outlined some internal structures (Fig. 2). The internal material consisted of rod-shaped structures which had a helical pattern. This helical material was released from completely disrupted particles and the nucleocapsid was shown to have a width of 150 to 180 Å with a central hole of approximately 50 Å diameter. The rod surface was serrated and had a periodicity of 50 to 60 Å (Fig. 3).

In earlier electron microscopic studies of CDV by REAGAN and BRUECKNER (1951), who used the metal shadowing technique, spherical particles were found with a mean diameter of 210 Å. It is now doubted that these particles represented the CD virion.

B. Physico-Chemical Structure

In comparison with other viruses, little is known about the physico-chemical structure of CD virus. More information is available on measles virus (NORRBY, 1967) which appears to be structurally and antigenically very similar to CDV. Two principal reasons have hampered more detailed work with CDV: It has not been possible to obtain high virus titers of CD virus in tissue culture and hemagglutination with CDV has not been found.

1. Type of Nucleic Acid

BUSSELL (1966) and KIMES and BUSSELL (1968) reported that cell cultures treated with the halogenated pyrimidine analogues, fluorodeoxyuridine and bromodeoxyuridine did not inhibit the production of infectious CDV. PHILLIPS and BUSSELL (1971 a) found 6-azauridine (0.025 mM) to inhibit 99 per cent of CDV formation whereas DNA containing vaccinia virus was only inhibited 20 per cent. Actinomycin D (0.01 μg/ml) caused only 23 per cent inhibition of CDV formation, whereas DNA containing herpes simplex virus was inhibited 99 per cent. All these metabolic inhibition studies strongly indicated the nucleic acid type of CDV to be RNA. Incorporation of radioactive labels into CDV nucleic acid was studied by PHILLIPS and BUSSELL (1971 a). They observed incorporation of ³H-uridine (2 mCi/ml), but ³H-thymidine (2 mCi/ml) was not incorporated. These data again left little doubt that CDV is a RNA virus.

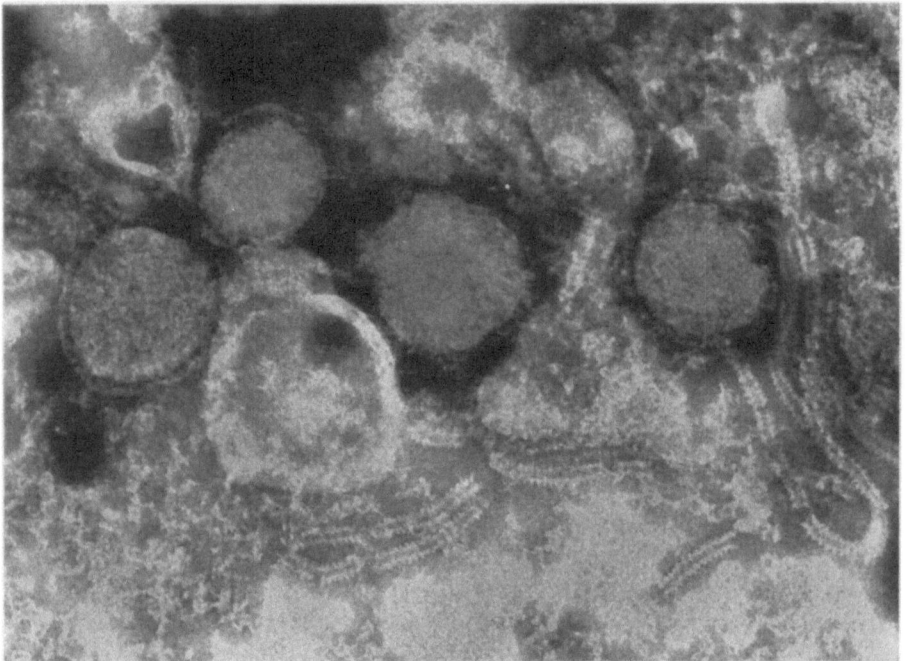

Fig. 1. Canine distemper virus negatively stained with phosphotungstate (× 180,000). Veterinary Virus Research Institute, Cornell University, Ithaca, New York 14850

2. Cytochemical Studies

HUNT et al. (1963) used various staining procedures to analyze the content of distemper inclusion bodies in cells. They found proteins or polypeptides characterized by the presence of the following reactive groups: histidine and cystine (sulf-hydryl groups), cystine (disulfide linkages), α-amino groups, tyrosine, arginine tryptophan, lysine, and glutamin. Purines and pyrimidines of nucleic acids may have been demonstrated. Lipids, carbohydrates, minerals, or DNA were not found. The authors assumed that inclusion bodies consisted of aggregates of viral particles, because MOULTON and BROWN (1954) had observed that distemper inclusions contained viral antigen, when stained with fluorescent antibody. The same observation was made by v. MICKWITZ and SCHRÖDER (1968). However, they found inclusions to persist longer than viral antigen. COFFIN and LIU (1957) found fuchsinophilic inclusions that stained with Seller's stain to contain viral antigen, while acidophilic inclusions stained with Shorr's tripple stain did not always contain antigen. It must be assumed that distemper inclusions are made of cellular material, which usually contains viral antigen. v. MICKWITZ and SCHRÖDER (1968) confirmed the cytochemical findings made by HUNT et al. (1963). In addition, they demonstrated RNA in inclusions with gallocyanin-chromalum, which could be neutralized with RNase digestion.

3. Buoyant Density

The mean buoyant density of the infectious CD virion was found to be essentially the same in cesium chloride (1.231 g/ml) and in potassium tartrate (1.233 g/ml) (PHILLIPS and BUSSELL, 1971 b). Three stable complement fixing antigens (CFA) banded in cesium chloride in different layers: A heavy CFA with a density of 1.289, probably a protein; a medium CFA in the range of infectious virus particles (1.234), probably lipoprotein; and a light CFA with a density of 1.140, probably a coat lipoprotein with a relatively high lipid content. Because CDV has a relatively low buoyant density in comparison with other viruses it can be assumed that it has a high percentage of protein and lipid material and a low percentage of nucleic acid. Continuous-flow ultracentrifugation banded infectious CDV between 32 and 48 per cent sucrose (ELLIOT and RYAN, 1970).

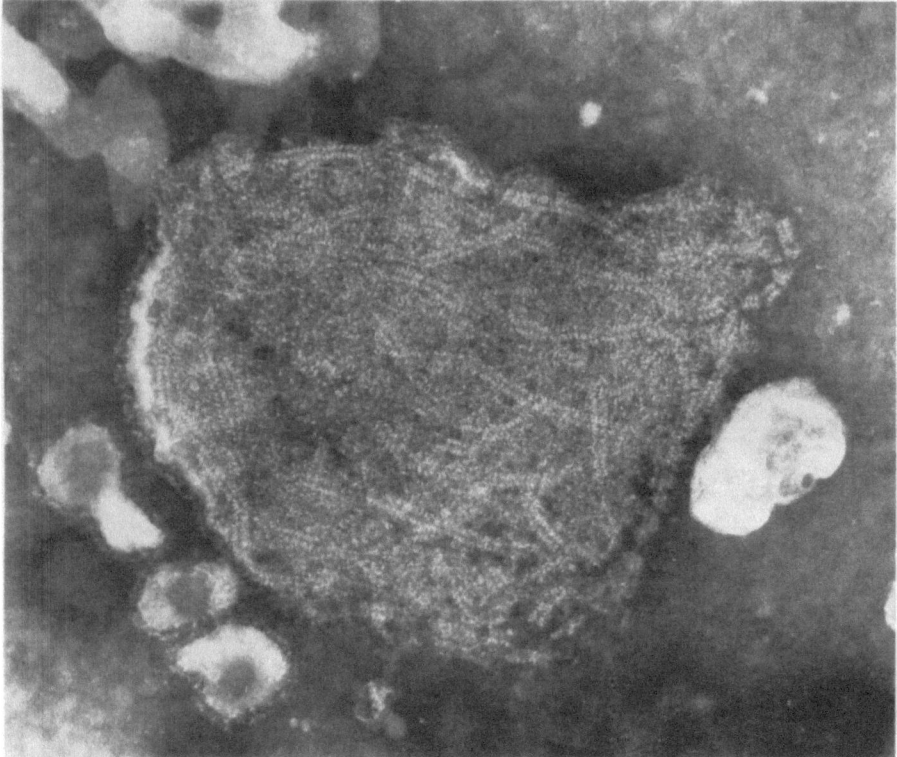

Fig. 2. Canine distemper virus negatively stained with phosphotungstate (× 150,000). Courtesy of J. D. ALMEIDA University of London, England

C. Antigenic Structure

Since structural antigens from fractionated CDV preparations have not been isolated and separated for serological tests, a direct relationship between antigenic structure and antibody response is not known. A number of studies give some indirect indication for the presence of V and S antigen in CDV. The structural and

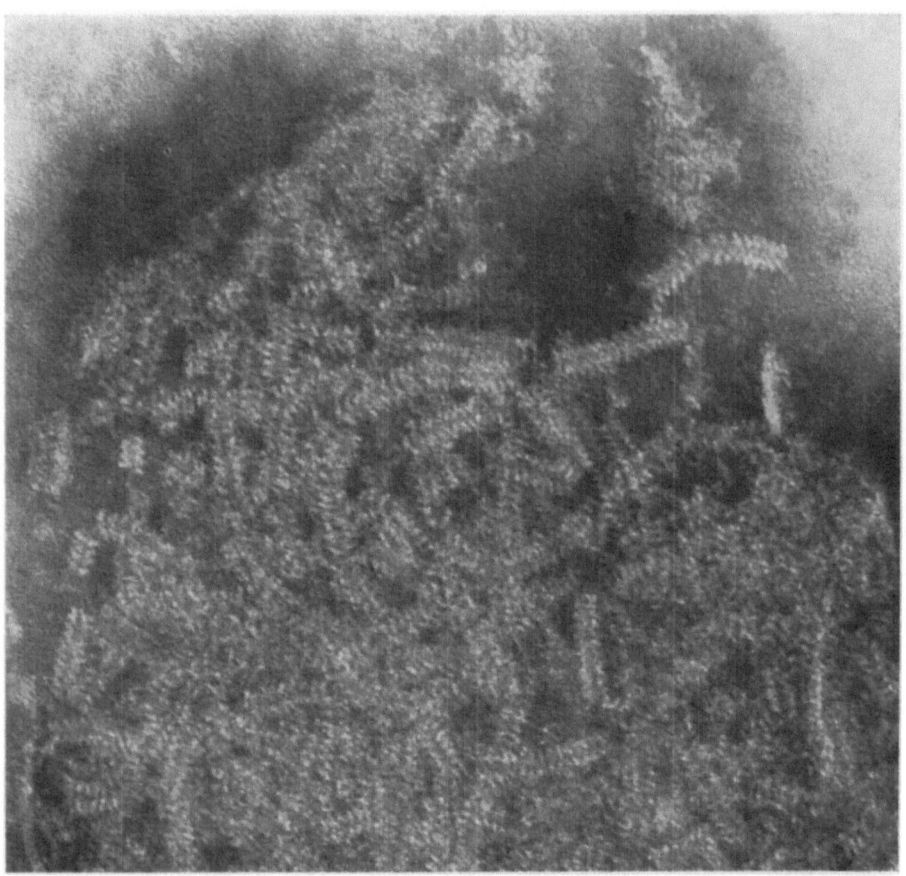

Fig. 3. Canine distemper virus negatively stained with phosphotungstate (× 250,000). Courtesy of J. D. ALMEIDA, University of London, England

antigenic relationship of CDV to measles virus permits the assumption of similar antigenic structure. However, hemagglutination has not been found with CDV. Obviously, more information is necessary for comparison.

Different isolates and various adapted strains of CDV cannot be differentiated serologically, like the other members of the MRD group. Common antigens and antibodies within this group will be discussed in the section on immunity.

In vitro serological tests which have been applied for the detection of antigens and antibody include complement fixation, agar gel diffusion precipitation, and fluorescent antibody studies.

1. Complement-Fixing Antigens

The complement fixation (CF) test with CDV has mainly been used as a diagnostic test, using a great variety of tissue suspensions from infected animals or embryonated hen eggs. Separation of various structural antigens from the distemper virion for comparison in CF tests have been made only recently (PHILLIPS and BUSSELL, 1971 b).

LAIDLAW and DUNKIN (1931) used spleen suspensions from infected ferrets in the CF reaction, employing an incubation period of 30 minutes at 37° C. Preincubation of the antigen for one hour at 50° C partially destroyed and for 30 minutes at 60° C completely destroyed the CF reaction. The heat-labile nature of CDV-CF antigen has been confirmed several times (MANSI, 1955). DRÄGER and SCHINDLER (1951) found CF antigen in saline suspensions of spleen, lymph nodes, tonsils, thymus, lung, salivary glands, pancreas, and urine from infected dogs. They used an incubation period of 16—18 hours at 6°—8° C. BINDRICH (1954) tested a similar range of tissues from infected dogs and ferrets and had best results with spleen and lymph nodes. Brain suspensions were useful from dogs with distemper encephalitis. DEDIE (1951) used 5 per cent tissue suspensions in saline; more concentrated material had anticomplementary effects. FASTIER (1956) eliminated anticomplementary reactions by ion exchange column chromatography. He used chorio-allantoic membrane (CAM) suspensions as antigen from infected embryonated hen eggs. A complement titration in addition to antigen titrations was considered necessary by MANSI (1955). In routine tests he used 4 to 6 units of complement. At least 5 different strains of CDV shared a common complement-fixing antigen in his study.

A soluble antigen that is separate from infectious particles and is heat-labile has been claimed by BINDRICH (1954) and MANSI (1955). However, their observation was based on the fact that CF negative tissue suspensions were still infectious when inoculated into dogs or ferrets, which was probably material with low virus titer.

PHILLIPS and BUSSELL (1971 b) separated 3 stable CF antigens by cesium chloride gradient centrifugation of CDV (Onderstepoort strain). One was probably a protein with a buoyant density of 1.289, the other two were probably lipoproteins with buoyant densities of 1.234 and 1.140.

2. Precipitating Antigen

MANSI (1957) used the agar-gel-diffusion test of Ouchterlony to study CDV. He used tissue fragments of mesenteric lymph node or spleen from infected animals as the source of antigen in a Petri dish system. Hyperimmune serum was placed into wells 0.4 cm distant from the antigen well. A single precipitin line was observed 24 hours later. Utilizing microscopic slides the system was made more sensitive and the precipitin line appeared in 1 to 3 hours as opposed to 5 to 18 hours in his plate test (MANSI, 1958).

WHITE and COWAN (1962) found soluble antigens distinct from the infective virus particles to precipitate with antibody in agar gel. The precipitating antigen was found in the supernatant fluid of infected tissue suspensions that had been centrifuged for 2 hours at $103,000 \times g$. It could be salted out from infected tissue culture fluids, and was inactivated at 56° C when heated for 30 minutes. On DEAE cellulose columns, the precipitating antigen was eluted with 0.25 M NaCl in phosphate buffer (pH 7.0), however, the bulk of infectivity was found in the 0.5 M NaCl eluate.

The electroprecipitin test for the detection of CDV was reported by ZYDECK (1970).

3. Immunofluorescent Antigens

The fluorescent antibody (FA) technique has been frequently used for demonstration of CD antigen in tissues and cells (MOULTON and BROWN, 1954; MOULTON, 1956; LIU and COFFIN, 1957; APPEL, 1969; BAUMANN, 1967; FAIRCHILD et al., 1967; SCHRÖDER et al., 1968). An attempt to label sites of formation of different antigens of CDV during a growth cycle has been made by YAMANOUCHI et al. (1970). They claimed V and S antigen both to be formed in the cytoplasm, since intranuclear fluorescence only appeared 48 or 72 hours after infection and a single growth cycle was approximately 18 hours (SHISHIDO et al., 1967). The authors used serum from convalescent dogs and assumed it to contain antibodies against both the V and S antigens. Complete virus on cell surfaces fluoresced, which indicated activity of the labelled serum against V antigen. However, activity against S antigen has not been shown.

4. Hemagglutination by CDV

VLADIMIROV (1949) has stated that CDV causes hemagglutination of human and frog erythrocytes at dilutions of 1 : 40 and 1 : 320. These results have not been confirmed. GORHAM (1960) failed to detect hemagglutination with the Onderstepoort egg-adapted strain and red blood cells from human type "0", rats, mice, guinea pigs, goats, rabbits, dogs, or ferrets. Utilizing the same viral strain in earlier studies HAIG (1949) observed irregular and partial agglutination of chicken and guinea pig erythrocytes. BUSSELL (personal communication) attempted monkey erythrocyte agglutination and hemolysis with CDV without success.

D. Resistance to Physical and Chemical Agents

1. Light

NEMO and CUTCHINS (1966) reported that CDV was inactivated by visible light. CUTCHINS and DAYHUFF (1962) had earlier reported that MV was similarly affected by visible light, consequently this effect on the CDV was anticipated by these investigators. CDV was light sensitive in fluid suspension as well as during intracellular replication. The addition of calf serum or glutathione reduced the rate of inactivation. The virus was less sensitive in distilled water. Amino acids and Earle's salts in minimal essential medium of Eagle had a stabilizing effect on light sensitivity but not vitamins or riboflavine. These findings showed that some ingredient of the medium may enhance light sensitivity but its presence is not necessary for light inactivation of CDV. The investigators postulated that some substance derived from the host cell and intimately associated with the virus particle serves to make it light sensitive.

2. Heat

Studies involving the response of virulent CDV to heat in various substrates, various viral concentrations, and with different isolates were made by several investigators. LAIDLAW and DUNKIN (1928 b) observed that virulent virus in dog spleen survives for 30 minutes at 60° C but not for 1 hour. BINDRICH (1954) found virulent virus in tissue suspension after 3 hours at 20° C, but a marked reduction after 15 hours. Virulent virus survived 37° C for 60 minutes, but was inactivated after 30 minutes at 56° C. GORHAM and BRANDLY (1953) showed virus in nasal exudate to survive for at least 20 minutes at room temperature. CELIKER and GILLESPIE (1954) found virus in suspended chorioallantoic membrane (CAM) inactivated in 10 minutes at 50° C. The infectious property of virus in the intact CAM was lost after 7 to 8 days at 25° C and after 7 to 8 weeks at 4° C. RECULARD *et al.* (1960) studied the effects of 15° C on virus in CAM suspension. There was no loss of virus after 1 hour but after 4 hours a 25 per cent loss, after 8 hours a 75 per cent loss, and after 15 hours complete inactivation occurred. There was also complete inactivation after 1 hour at 37° C.

BUSSELL and KARZON (1962) studied the heat inactivation kinetics on CDV in chick-embryo cell culture. The viral half-life was 120 minutes at 21° C, 60 minutes at 37° C, 10 minutes at 45° C, and 2 to 3 minutes at 56° C. Lo *et al.* (1965 a) had similar results with avianized CDV in eggs.

3. Low Temperature

Storage at low temperatures is a satisfactory way to preserve CDV. Many investigators have noticed that holding the virus above 0° C resulted in rather quick destruction, and freezing and thawing of CDV caused a reduction in titer. GORHAM (1960) reported that the Onderstepoort strain of CDV had remained viable in infected CAM for 37 months at −16° to −18° C, and in a 10 per cent suspension for at least 60 days at −5° C. Infected ferret spleens retained their pathogenicity for ferrets after storage for 693 days at −24° C (GORHAM, 1960). Infectivity of virus in tissue suspensions remained for at least 172 days at −30° C (BINDRICH, 1954). There was no loss of chick embryo cell propagated virus 2 and 8 days after storage at −30° C, but a 50 per cent occurred after 6 months (RECULARD *et al.*, 1960). Egg-adapted virus, either Lederle or Onderstepoort strains, suspended in sucrose-glucose-glutamate solution as 1 : 3 suspension, retained the infective titer for at least 6 months at −65° C (GILLESPIE, unpublished). CDV propagated in embryonated hens' eggs and stored in pieces of infected CAM remained viable for at least 7 years at −65° C (GILLESPIE, unpublished). Similar results were obtained with infective dog spleen and brain.

4. Lyophilization

This method provides another way to preserve CDV in the laboratory and for commercial use. Lyophilizers which apply heat to remove residual moisture from egg-adapted strains cause a significant loss of titer, usually from 0.5 to 1.5 $\log_{10}$ of virus. This may be critical for a commercial vaccine product depending upon its titer prior to lyophilization and subsequent treatment after reconstitution with sterile distilled water. Lyophilized CDV is very stable, either as virulent or modified virus, if the moisture content is low enough. Using glass sealed ampoules under nitrogen, SIEDENTOPF and GREEN (1942) maintained ferret-adapted virus (Distemperiod) for 365 days at 7° C. BINDRICH (1954) kept lyophilized CD for 5 months at 5° C without loss of infectivity. GORHAM (1960) also had favorable results with this procedure. The Wisconsin FXNO strain was viable for at least 7 years at 5° to 7° C.

5. pH Stability

BINDRICH (1951 c) reported that CDV is comparatively resistant to pH 4.5 and above. It was partially inactivated at pH 9 and completely inactivated at a higher pH when maintained at 5° C for 30 minutes. He concluded that the optimal pH for CVD was pH 7. CELIKER and GILLESPIE (1954) reported on the survival of the Onderstepoort strain at various pH levels. Viability was retained between values of 4.4 and 10.4; at higher and lower values infectivity was lost. Maximal stability of the Wisconsin FXNO strain was obtained at pH 8.8 while viral activity declined above pH 9 and below pH 8 (DICKSON et al., 1955).

6. Radiation Effects

PALM and BLACK (1961 b) showed that CDV is inactivated by ultraviolet light at the rate of 1.0 log unit per 22,000 ergs per cm². Irradiation with 10^5 roentgens of gamma particles reduced the titer 0.4 log units at $-70°$ C and 1 log unit at 0° C.

7. Chemical Agents

Like other members of the myxovirus and paramyxovirus group, CDV is inactivated by chloroform and ether. BINDRICH and SCHMIDT (1955) worked with two strains of CDV in suspension. The Greifswald isolate retained its antigenicity in the CF test but lost its infectivity after a 15 minute treatment with chloroform. The Berlin virus, however, retained its infectivity and antigenicity when held under similar conditions by these same investigators. A 0.3 solution of chloroform inactivated the egg-adapted viral suspension after exposure at 4° C for 10 minutes. It is generally agreed that CDV is not infective when the virus is maintained for a sufficient period of time in an adequate concentration of ether or chloroform (PALM and BLACK, 1961 b). BINDRICH (1954) reported inactivation of CDV by ether and chloroform, but not by acetone.

Only limited information exists on the effects of formalin on CDV despite the fact that this chemical has been used for many years to produce an inactivated vaccine. Most of the studies were conducted with a 20 per cent suspension of infective ferret spleen. LAIDLAW and DUNKIN (1928 b) used 0.25 per cent formalin at 5° C for 24 hours to inactivate ferret virus. PINKERTON (1940) recommended 0.3 per cent formalin at 5° C for 4 days prior to use as a vaccine. HUMMON and BUSHNELL (1943) felt that the procedure used by PINKERTON was inadequate to inactivate the ferret viral suspension. They suggested an inactivation period for 7 days at 5° C. WEST and BRANDLY (1949) used 0.5 per cent formalin for inactivation and held the mixture at 6° C for 7 days before use as a vaccine. BINDRICH (1954) reported that virulent virus was inactivated by 0.05 per cent formalin at 37° C for 4 hours. In a suspension of infective CAM, egg-adapted CDV was inactivated after exposure to 0.1 per cent at 4° C for 1 to 2 hours. CELIKER and GILLESPIE (1954) also showed that 0.225 per cent formalin caused viral inactivation after exposure for 10 to 20 minutes at 4° C.

Two other chemicals studied by CELIKER and GILLESPIE (1954) for their virucidal effects were phenol and Roccal; the latter a commonly used quarternary ammonium disinfectant. A 0.75 per cent solution of phenol inactivated egg virus in 10 minutes at 4° C. Roccal inactivated the same virus at a concentration of 0.2 per cent after 30 minutes at 4° C while 0.3 per cent permitted the same result within 10 minutes at 4° C.

Hydroxylamine inactivated CDV (KIMES and BUSSELL, 1968), however, different conditions may change results (BUSSELL, personal communication).

Beta-propiolactone in a final concentration of 0.1 per cent inactivated CDV within 2 hours at 37° C (BUSSELL, personal communication).

E. Cultivation

1. History

The first reported attempt to propagate virulent CDV in tissue culture came from MITSCHERLICH (1938). Using the plasma-clot method with small pieces of spleen or lung in a drop of dog plasma on coverslips, he observed growth of fibroblasts around tissue pieces but no cytopathic effect (CPE). Distemper could be transmitted to dogs with culture fluids taken a few days after inoculation of virus but not thereafter. DEDIE and KLAPÖTKE (1951, 1952) infected minced pieces of spleen, mesenteric lymph nodes, lung, and testes from 10-to-14-week old dogs with virulent CDV and found viral replication by animal inoculation up to 10 days of cultivation. CDV was serially passaged 19 times in spleen cultures and virus titers reached 2×10^4 log infectious doses per gram of tissue. Using mouse embryo brain explants (KLAPÖTKE, 1953), CDV titers were even higher. Twenty six passages were made successfully and the 18th passage was adapted to adult white mouse brain. Minced chicken embryos (LASFARGUES, 1953), ferret kidney, ferret trachea, and dog lung (HOPPER, 1959) in plasma clot roller culture infected with CDV gave similar results. HOPPER (1959) also found HeLa cells and a human liver cell line to support CDV through 2 passages and a total of 24 days cultivation without any obvious CPE.

2. Host Cell Range

Isolation of virulent canine distemper virus (CDV) in tissue culture is difficult, however, it has been achieved by several investigators in various cell systems (Table 1). Once adapted to embryonating chicken eggs or tissue culture, the virus can be propagated in a large number of cell types from different species. CDV has been adapted to canine, mustelid, avian, bovine, simian, and human cell cultures (Table 2). Primary cell cultures as well as cell lines have been employed for adaptation. Epithelial and fibroblastic cultures are susceptible for adaptation once the initial infection has been achieved. Dog kidney, chick embryo fibroblast, and green monkey kidney monolayer cell cultures most commonly have been used for experimental work and vaccine production.

Since the host cell range of virulent CDV differs from the host cell range of adapted CDV, they will be discussed in separate sections:

a) Virulent Virus

In spite of many attempts, relatively few reports have been made on the propagation of virulent CDV in tissue culture. One explanation may be that the primary target cells of CDV *in vivo* appear to be macrophages and cells from lymphatic tissues (LIU and COFFIN, 1957; APPEL, 1969) while attempts to grow CDV have been made mainly in epithelial and fibroblastic type cells.

Table 1. *Host-Cell Range of Virulent Canine Distemper Virus in Cell Cultures*

Cell Type	Virus Growth	CPE	Reference
I. Dog			
1. Primary monolayer cultures			
Kidney	+	+	ROCKBORN, 1958 a
Lung	+	+	VANTSIS, 1959
Lung macrophages	+	+	APPEL and JONES, 1967
Brain	+	+	GIBSON, 1968
Cerebellar explants	+	+	STORTS et al., 1968
2. Primary suspension cultures			
Lymphocytes	+	−	POSTE, 1970
3. Continuous cultures			
Melanoma	+	+	KASZA and GRIESEMER, 1967
Thyroidal carcinoma	+	+	KASZA and GRIESEMER, 1967
Bladder carcinoma	+	+	APPEL, unpublished
II. Ferret			
1. Primary kidney	+	+	VANTSIS, 1959
2. Macrophages	+	+	POSTE, 1971

ROCKBORN (1958 a) succeeded in propagating virulent CDV in dog kidney (DK) cell cultures. He used serum from infected dogs to inoculate monolayer cultures of primary DK cells. Forty-two days after inoculation he observed generalized cytoplasmic degeneration and vacuolization of cells. Although CPE occurred much earlier after further passages, and his finding was a major breakthrough for adaptation of CDV to tissue culture and for vaccine production, susceptibility of DK cells for virulent CDV was too low for isolation purposes. BITTLE *et al.* (1961) confirmed Rockborn's results by adapting virulent CDV from a dog spleen suspension to DK cultures. By keeping cultures on roller drums they first observed CPE 18 days after inoculation (Fig. 9); adaptation with further passage occurred rapidly.

VANTSIS (1959) and CORNWELL *et al.* (1965) prepared lung and kidney monolayer cell cultures from dogs and ferrets for isolation of virulent CDV. Ferret kidney cell cultures were found by these authors to be most susceptible. This observation has not been confirmed by other groups (HOPPER, 1959; HARRISON, 1968 a).

Canine melanoma, canine thyroidal carcinoma (KASZA and GRIESEMER, 1967), and canine bladder carcinoma (APPEL, unpublished) cell lines proved to be susceptible to virulent CDV. These cells were not susceptible enough for routine virus isolation and CPE occurred late and slowly. Canine brain monolayer cultures (GIBSON, 1968) gave similar results. Cerebellar explants from newborn dogs sup-

Table 2. *Host-Cell Range of Attenuated Canine Distemper Virus in Cell Cultures*

Cell Type	Virus Growth	CPE	Reference
I. Canine			
1. Primary cultures			
Kidney	+	+	ROCKBORN, 1958 a
Lung macrophages	+	+	APPEL, 1967
Lymphocytes	+	−	POSTE, 1970
2. Continuous cultures			
Kidney (MDCK)	+	+	IMAGAWA et al., 1963
Melanoma	+	+	KASZA and GRIESEMER, 1967
Thyroidal carcinoma	+	+	KASZA and GRIESEMER, 1967
II. Ferret			
Primary kidney	+	+	SHAVER et al., 1964
Macrophages	+	+	POSTE, 1971
III. Avian			
Primary embryonic fibroblasts	+	−	CABASSO et al., 1959
IV. Bovine			
Primary kidney	+	+	BUSSEL and KARZON, 1965 b
V. Simian			
1. Primary cultures			
Rhesus kidney	+	+	BUSSEL and KARZON, 1965 b
Tamarian kidney	+	+	BUSSEL and KARZON, 1965 b
2. Continuous cultures			
Rhesus kidney (LLC-MK$_2$)	+	+	BUSSEL and KARZON, 1965 b
Green monkey kidney (CGM)	+	+	BUSSEL and KARZON, 1965 b
Green monkey kidney (Vero)	+	+	SHISHIDO et al., 1967
Green monkey kidney (BS-C-1)	+	+	HARRISON, 1964
VI. Human			
1. Primary cultures			
Amnion	+	+	BUSSEL and KARZON, 1965 b
2. Continuous cultures			
Amnion (AV$_3$, WS)	+	+	BUSSEL and KARZON, 1965 b
Fibroblasts (HLP)	+	+	BUSSEL and KARZON, 1965 b
HeLa	+	+	HOPPER, 1959
HEp-2	+	+	BUSSELL, pers. commun.

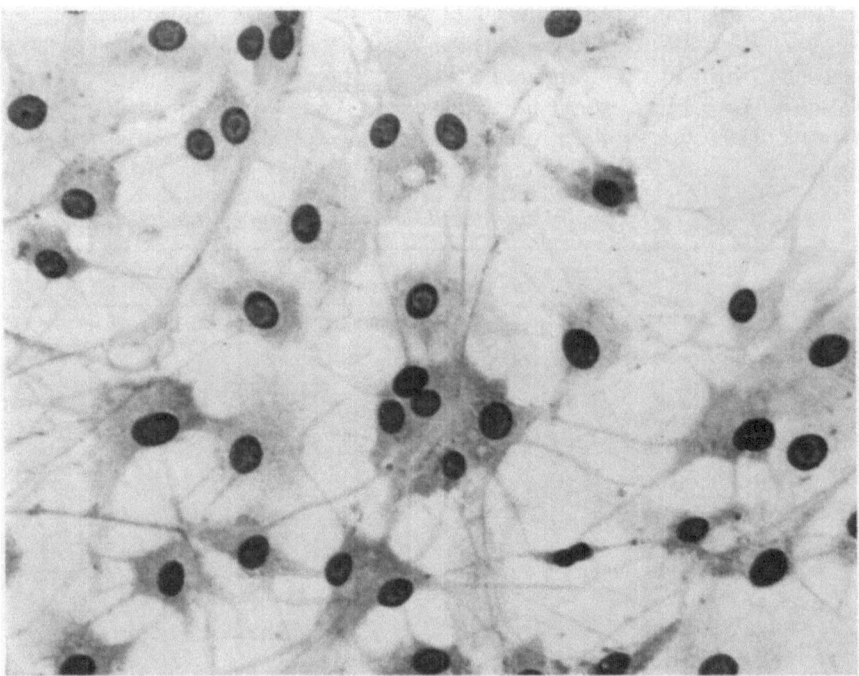

Fig. 5. Effect of canine distemper virus on explant tissue culture of canine cerebellum. Fifty-seven-day-old culture (52 days post-inoculation) showing the marked intranuclear inclusion body formation in astroglia located in the outgrowth. May-Grünwald-Giemsa stain (× 315). Reprinted with permission from: Storts *et al.*, Acta neuropath. (Berl.) **11**, 8 (1968)

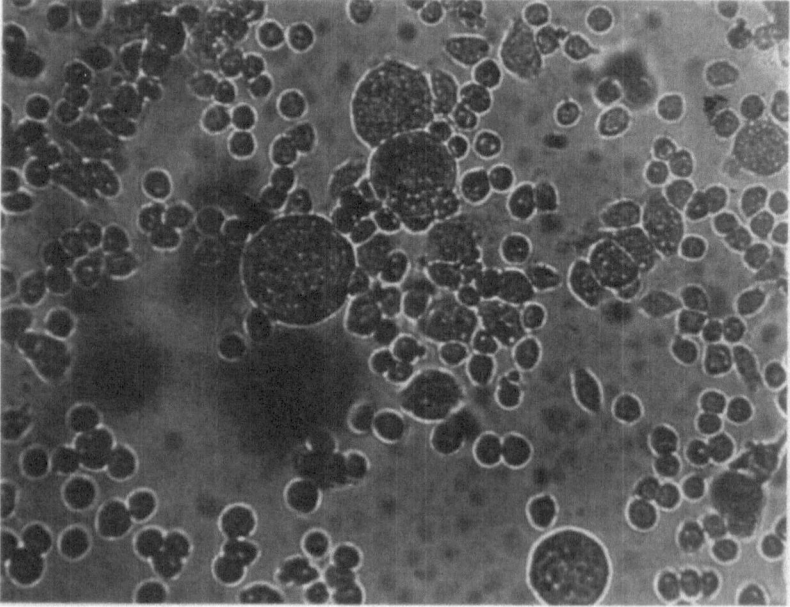

Fig. 6. Multinucleated giant cell formation in dog alveolar macrophage cultures 3 days after inoculation with virulent CD virus. Unstained (× 100)

ported growth of virulent virus (STORTS *et al.*, 1968). Explants were inoculated after 4 to 7 days of growth. Large polygonal astroglia and fusiform mesenchymal cells in peripheral outgrowth surrounding explants were first affected (Figs. 4, 5).

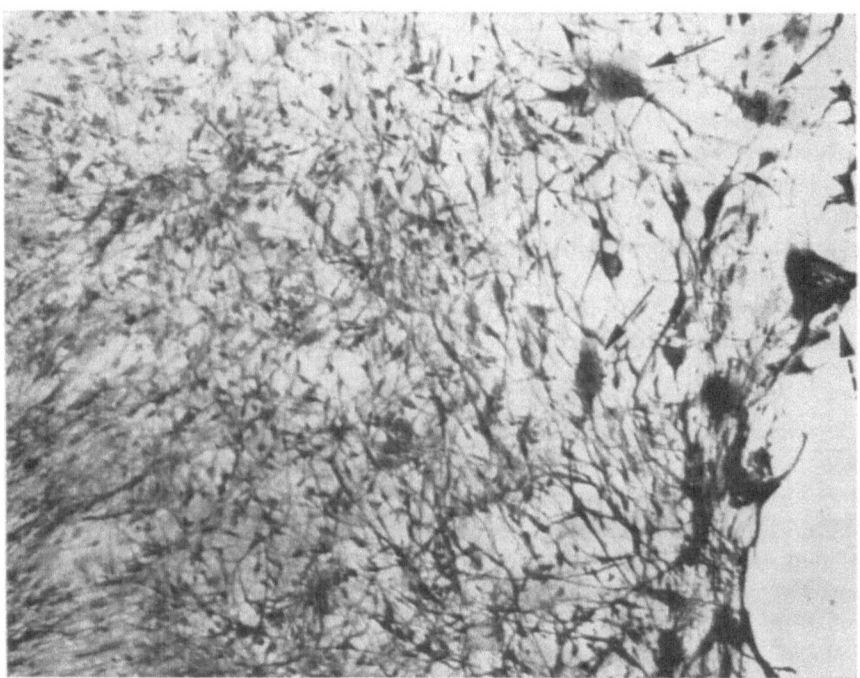

Fig. 4. Effect of canine distemper virus on explant tissue culture of canine cerebellum. Forty-three-day-old culture (36 days post-inoculation) demonstrating the reticulated pattern detected in infected cultures. Holmes' silver impregnation (× 50). Several syncytial formations can be seen in the outgrowth (arrows) with a contracted, degenerated one also present (broken arrow). The fibrous astrocytes throughout the outer threefourths of the outgrowth have contracted perikarya and prominent processes. Reprinted with permission from: STORTS *et al.*, Acta neuropath. (Berl.) 11, 7 (1968)

APPEL and JONES (1967) used dog alveolar macrophages to propagate virulent CDV. Macrophages were obtained by stirring minced lung pieces from SPF dogs in tissue culture medium without trypsin to separate alveolar macrophages. Virulent virus from several strains as well as from natural cases of distemper was inoculated into macrophage cultures shortly after seeding. Multinucleated giant-cell formation (Fig. 6) was noticed 2 to 5 days after inoculation, depending upon the titer of virus inoculated. Virus replication was shown in serial passages. This method was suitable for titration of virulent distemper virus and the titers obtained in macrophage cultures were similar to virus titrations in dogs. Viral growth associated with giant-cell formation was also found with cells obtained from bronchial washings of dogs with acute distemper that were placed in tissue culture medium. Similar results were reported by POSTE (1971). Polykariocytosis was induced by CDV in macrophages from lung, liver, spleen and peritoneum of dog and ferret origin.

Suspension cultures of dog lymphocytes supported growth of virulent CDV (POSTE, 1970). When cultures were treated with heterologous antilymphocyte serum, virus titers increased 80-fold within 3 days after inoculation. The increase in virus titers was directly related to an increase in number of lymphoblasts present in these cultures.

Another technique for isolating virulent CDV from infected animals is culti-vation of infected tissues. This method was used by VANTSIS (1959) who prepared monolayer cell cultures of kidney and lung tissue from CDV infected ferrets and dogs and found syncytia formation 6 or 7 days after seeding. BUSSELL and KARZON (1965 a) had similar results. Adaptation of virulent virus to tissue culture has been achieved using this method. HARRISON et al. (1968 a) infected ferrets with the CSL (Com-monwealth Serum Laboratories) strain of virulent CDV and prepared kidney monolayer cultures from an infected ferret. Passages were made at 14 day inter-vals into newly seeded normal ferret kidney (FK) cell cultures. All earlier attempts by the authors had failed to passage CDV in FK monolayer cell cultures from normal ferrets. KASZA (1968), THIEL et al. (1968), and SMITH et al. (1970) used this technique to isolate CDV from stray dogs without clinical distemper, which either reflected persistent virus or presence of virus during the incubation period.

b) Adapted Virus

Canine distemper virus was first adapted to embryonated hen eggs [HAIG, 1948; CABASSO and COX, 1949 (cf. p. 30)], and to dog kidney (DK) cell culture (ROCKBORN, 1958 a). These original adapted strains of CDV as well as later adap-ted strains have been used for a great number of subpassages and adaptation to different cell systems from several different species (Table 2). There is no ex-planation available why adapted virus is easier to passage to different cell systems from different species than virulent virus. A great variety of conditions have been employed in the propagation of adapted CDV in cell cultures. Results, therefore, are difficult to compare.

Dog kidney cells (ROCKBORN, 1958 a, 1959, 1960; VANTSIS, 1959; BITTLE et al., 1961; IMAGAWA et al., 1963; BUSSELL and KARZON, 1965 a; HARRISON et al., 1968 a), chick embryo fibroblasts (CABASSO et al., 1959; KARZON and BUSSELL, 1959; RECULARD, 1960) and green monkey kidney cell lines (HARRISON, 1964; BUSSELL and KARZON, 1965 b; SHISHIDO et al., 1967) are the most commonly used cell cultures for the propagation of adapted CDV. The VERO cells (SHISHIDO et al., 1967) attracted much attention recently, since most CDV strains can be adapted and avianized strains cause CPE without adaptation. They appear prom-ising for plaquing and plaque reduction tests (GOURLAY, 1970) and for serum neutralization tests (BROWN, personal communication; APPEL, unpublished). Ferret kidney cells are susceptible to a variety of adapted CDV strains (HOPPER, 1959; SHAVER, 1964; BUSSELL and KARZON, 1965 a). Mink kidney cells were used for adapted CDV vaccine production (ACKERMANN, 1968). Bovine kidney cells, human amnion cells in primary (Fig. 7) and continuous culture, a human fibro-blast cell line (BUSSELL and KARZON, 1965 b), a human liver cell line and HeLa cells (HOPPER, 1959), canine melanoma and thyroidal carcinoma cell lines (KASZA and GRIESEMER, 1967) were all susceptible for adapted CDV. Dog and ferret macrophages formed polykariocytosis and replicated attenuated CDV (APPEL, 1967, POSTE, 1971). Dog lymphocyte suspension cultures supported growth of adapted CDV and virus titers increased after treatment with antilymphocyte serum (POSTE, 1970).

Adapted CDV probably has a much wider cell host range. Frequent fluid changes, inoculation of young cells, maintenance of cell cultures on roller drums all improve conditions for adaptations and better virus titers. Infected macrophages or buffy coat cells can be overlayed on epithelial or fibroblastic monolayer cultures and foci of infected monolayer cells can be observed with fluorescent antibody a few days later (APPEL, unpublished).

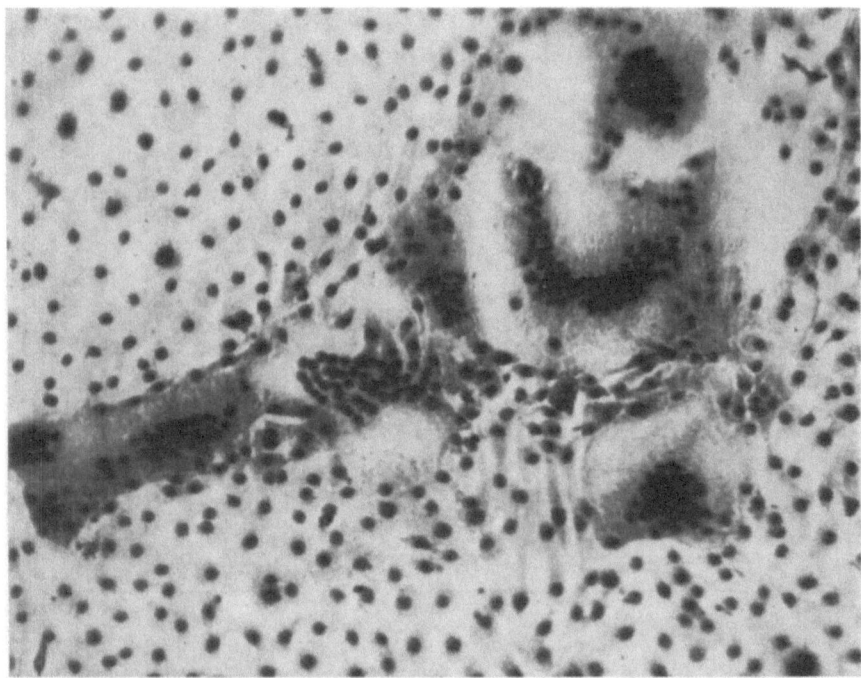

Fig. 7. Strain 4856 of CDV in primary human amnion cells, day 21. Focal syncytia ($\times$ 100). Reprinted with permission from: BUSSELL and KARZON, Arch. ges. Virusforsch. **17**, 183, (1965)

3. Virus Multiplication in Tissue Culture

a) Adsorption

Adsorption time of CDV to cells was only reported by BUSSELL and KARZON (1962). They inoculated chicken embryo fibroblast monolayer (CEF) cultures with the Onderstepoort strain that had been propagated in CEF cultures. Medium was removed at 15-minute intervalls, cultures were washed three times with PBS and were overlaid with agar. Plaque formation was used as an indicator for the amount of virus adsorbed. In four experiments, 50 per cent of the virus was adsorbed by 30 minutes and 4 hours were required for maximal adsorption. In two additional experiments, maximum adsorption was obtained at 2 hours.

b) Growth Curves

Growth curves for CDV were made by BUSSELL and KARZON (1962) with the Onderstepoort strain in CEF cultures and by SHISHIDO et al. (1967) with the CEF adapted Lederle strain in an African green monkey kidney cell line (Vero cells)

(Fig. 8). BUSSELL and KARZON adsorbed virus at an input ratio of 1 : 1 (virus : cells) for 1 to 2 hours and incubated at 36° C. After an eclipse phase of 8 to 10 hours virus appeared in the cells; after 10 to 13 hours it was found in the supernatant fluid. Virus yields then increased logarithmically at a rate of approximately 0.3 log per hour until 18 hours. There was a distinct plateau in both the supernatant and the cell-associated virus, which occurred between 17 and 24 hours. This time probably represented the end of one complete growth cycle. Peak virus titers reached 10^6 plaque forming units (PFU)/ml as cell-associated virus and $10^{4.5}$ PFU/ml in the supernatant between 30 and 60 hours.

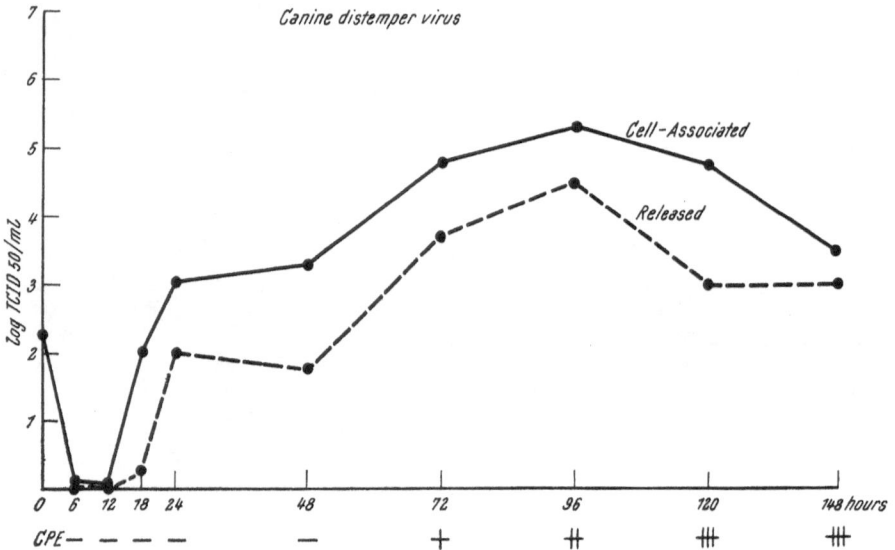

Fig. 8. Growth curve of canine distemper virus in Vero cells. Virus was inoculated at an input multiplicity of 0.3.
Reprinted with permission from: SHISHIDO et al., Arch. ges. Virusforsch. 22, 375 (1967)

SHISHIDO et al. (1967) adsorbed virus at an input ratio of 1 : 3 for 1 hour in roller drums at 37° C. The eclipse period before appearance of cell-associated virus was 12 to 18 hours. Release of virus into supernatant fluid was first noted at 18 hours. The maximum infectivity titer of cell associated virus was $10^{5.3}$ TCID$_{50}$ per ml and supernatant virus was $10^{4.5}$ TCID$_{50}$ per ml between 72 to 96 hours. Infectivity titers of released virus never exceeded that of cell-associated virus.

4. Cytopathic Effects

Canine distemper virus which replicates in tissue culture usually produces cytopathic effects (CPE), sometimes only after several passages. They consist mostly of multinucleated giant cell (syncytia) formation, and intracytoplasmic and intranuclear inclusion bodies. Syncytia usually, but not always, can be seen in unstained preparations under the light microscope. They vary from small, round, or stellate type forms, with only several nuclei, to large masses of nuclei packed together, surrounded by cytoplasm. Inclusion bodies are only visible in stained preparations. Degeneration of cells, such as granular appearance of cytoplasm and vacuolization and detaching of cells, can usually be observed. Foci of CPE first appear anywhere in the cell sheet. In some cell systems the CPE remains restricted to foci, but in most cases CPE generalizes and spreads out from the initial foci. Time and intensity of the occurrence of CPE varies greatly between different strains of virus, different types of cells, different media, and incubation conditions. Young cells are always more susceptible and produce CPE more readily than older cells. Cytopathic effects and virus titers appear to be higher in rolled than in stationary cultures. Frequent fluid changes and maintenance of the pH level at 7.2 to 7.6 increase CPE and total virus yield. The optimal temperature appears to be 35° to 36° C.

When ROCKBORN (1958 a) first adapted virulent CDV to primary dog kidney (DK) cells he noticed the first CPE 42 days postinfection (PI). His monolayers were inoculated with serum from infected dogs. After 8 passages time of appearance of CPE was reduced to 2 days. Scattered foci of smaller cells with unusual granular structure of the cytoplasm appeared first, followed the next day by vacuoles in some cells and the appearance of syncytia. Two days later giant cells were numerous, some containing 50 or more nuclei. Eosinophilic inclusion bodies were found in stained preparations. BITTLE et al. (1961) reported similar results. After 21 passages of virulent CDV in DK cultures giant cells and intracytoplasmic inclusion bodies (Fig. 9) appeared 7 days PI, intranuclear inclusions were seen only 3 days later. The occurrence of intranuclear inclusion bodies a few days after the appearance of intracytoplasmic inclusions is stated in most reports on CDV in tissue culture. Inclusion bodies, especially intracytoplasmic, tend to appear

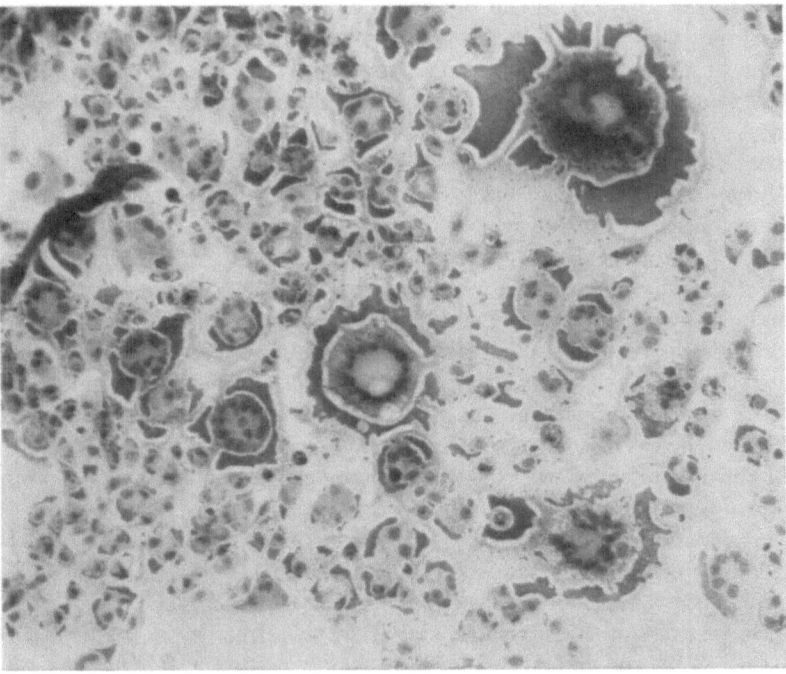

Fig. 9. Canine kidney tissue culture 16 days after infection with 6th tissue culture passage distemper virus. Note cytoplasmic inclusions and syncytia. Phloxine-tartrazine (× 120). Reprinted with permission from: BITTLE et al., Cornell Vet. 51, 365 (1961)

first as fine granules which become larger and fuse several days later to large homogenous masses involving the entire cytoplasm of single cells or of giant cells.

Cytopathic changes in primary ferret kidney (FK) cells are similar to CPE in DK cells. Intranuclear inclusions were rare with the Onderstepoort egg-adapted strain but not with the Rockborn DK-adapted strain (SHAVER, 1964). Virus yields with the Rockborn strain were less in FK cells than in DK cells (BUSSELL and KARZON, 1965 a). Cytopathic effects were less pronounced with egg-adapted strains.

Chick embryo fibroblast (CEF) cultures tend to produce less CPE than epithelial type monolayer cultures. In spite of 64 serial passages with virus titers ranging from 10^3 to $10^{4.5}$ EID$_{50}$ per ml, CABASSO et al. (1959) did not observe CPE with the Lederle strain of CDV. KARZON and BUSSELL (1959) observed granular appearance of cytoplasm, rounding and fragmentation of cells, but no evidence of syncytial formation with both the Lederle and Onderstepoort strains of egg-adapted CDV. They grew CEF cells in Earle's salt solution with calf serum. However, when cells were grown with horse serum and maintained in 199 medium as described by CABASSO, only the Onderstepoort strain was cytopathic. This is a good example for the influence of various conditions of CPE. Intracytoplasmic and intranuclear inclusions were seen in CEF cells with avianized CDV (RECULARD et al., 1960).

Cytopathic effects in monkey kidney (MK) cells, primary or continuous, tend to be similar to CPE in DK cells, however, are often not as extensive. The Onderstepoort strain and strain 4856 (BUSSELL and KARZON, 1965 b) produced syncytia and inclusions in rhesus and Tamarian primary kidney cells between 5 and 18 days PI. In LLC-MK$_2$ and CGM cell lines syncytia were found with the Onderstepoort strain after propagation in AV 3 cells. When grown in CEF cells, CPE induction in MK cell lines was slower but stellate type degeneration appeared in addition to syncytial formation. Virus yields ranged from $10^{3.2}$ to $10^{4.7}$ TCID$_{50}$ per ml.

When HARRISON (1964, 1968) first attempted CDV adaptation to BS-C-1 cells, a diploid epithelial cell line from green monkey kidneys, passages at 7 day intervals were unsuccessful. However, at 14 day intervals she succeeded; virus titers and CPE came to a peak (10^5 to 10^6 TCID$_{50}$ per ml) 9 to 12 days PI.

In Vero green monkey kidney cells (SHISHIDO, 1967), syncytia and inclusions were found 5 days PI with the Lederle strain, and 11 days PI with the Wisconsin and Onderstepoort strain of CDV. After serial passages, CPE with all strains appeared 3 to 5 days PI. Granulation and vacuolation became prominent 1 or 2 days after the first appearance of giant cells. Eventually cells degenerated and became detached. Virus titers reached 10^5 TCID$_{50}$ per ml.

Cell cultures infected with CDV sometimes can be maintained for prolonged times inspite of extensive CPE and constant virus release. IMAGAWA et al. (1963) found persisting virus titers of 10^4 to $10^{4.5}$ per ml for 15 weeks in the Madin-Darby canine kidney cell line infected with the Rockborn strain. Cytoplasmic and intranuclear inclusions and multinucleated giant cells were abundant.

Slowly progressing CPE with Snyder Hill and ferret origin strains of CDV in canine melanoma and canine thyroidal carcinoma cell lines were found by KASZA and GRIESEMER (1967). Giant cells first appeared 8 to 15 days PI; cytoplasmic and intranuclear inclusions 14 to 21 days PI. After 20 additional days CPE became more prominent. Complete cellular degeneration occurred after 40 to 50 days PI in the thyroid cell line. It occurred even later in the melanoma cell line, where many cells remained unaffected up to 120 days PI. A similar observation was made with the Snyder Hill strain in a canine urinary bladder carcinoma cell line (APPEL, unpublished).

In a search for a demyelination model, STORTS et al. (1968) infected cerebellar explants from newborn dogs with virulent CDV. Virus, that had been passaged 3 times in brain monolayer cultures, induced small, granular intracytoplasmic inclusion bodies in astroglia and mesenchymal cells 8 days postinoculation. Inclusions became larger by the 10th and 12th day and syncytial giant cells were formed by both cell types (Fig. 4). By the 15th day astrocytic growth had replaced most of the mesenchymal cells and giant cells were abundant. Intranuclear inclusions were noticed in astroglia (Fig. 5). Intracytoplasmic and intranuclear inclusion bodies were seen to contain viral antigen when labelled with fluorescent antibody. In spite of some degeneration and necrosis in explants and outgrowth, several cultures were maintained for 52 days postinoculation without extensive cell destruction. Degeneration of neurons and their processes was first seen in large neurons 3 to 4 weeks postinoculation, when the same cells in uninoculated control cultures were still intact. Degeneration of granule and stellate cells was also noticed. Intranuclear inclusions were seen in granule cells. Cultures that were inoculated with CDV either failed to myelinate or demyelinated shortly after the development of myelin sheath. Myelinated axons became irregular, the sheath disrupted and dissolved approximately 1 week before detectable neuronal changes were noticed.

5. Cell Fusion Factor

A cell fusion factor (CFF) has been repeatedly found in paramyxoviruses and has been demonstrated in measles virus by CASCARDO and KARZON (1965). The CFF was still present in inactivated virus preparations. BUSSELL (personal communication) observed cell fusion and syncytial formation in tissue culture cells several hours after inoculation with unfrozen CDV (Onderstepoort strain) but only several days after inoculation with frozen CDV. However, when CDV infected whole cells were frozen with glycerol to keep cells intact, and virus from these cells was passaged, cell fusion again occurred quickly. He concluded that the CFF depended on intact cells. It was still present in beta-propiolactone inactivated CDV.

6. Plaque Formation

Plaque formation in tissue culture induced by CDV has been demonstrated by BUSSELL and KARZON (1962, 1965 a), HARRISON et al. (1968), and GOURLAY (1970). BUSSELL and KARZON (1962) used primary chick embryo cell cultures prepared from 10-to-11-day old chick embryos. Cultured cells were inoculated with virus dilutions 24 to 48 hours after seeding of cells, when confluent monolayers had formed. The Onderstepoort and Lederle strains, and strains 4856 were used for inoculation. They had been propagated in chick embryo cells, on the CAM of chicken embryos, or in ferret kidney cells. After a 30-minute adsorption period at 36° C the cultures were overlaid with agar medium. Plaques were counted after an 11-day incubation period at 36° C. The Onderstepoort strain induced plaques within 4 or 5 days inoculation while the Lederle strain and strain 4856 required 7 to 9 days. On the 11th day plaques reached an average size of 2 mm with the Onderstepoort strain and between 0.5 to 1 mm with the other strains. Plaque formation began with rounding of cells and a granular appearance, which later was seen as condensed-cell debris, with areas free of cells. A linear relationship between virus concentration and plaque number was demonstrated.

Using AV 3 cells and the Onderstepoort strain for plaque induction, Bussell and Karzon (1965 a) employed their original methods. Plaques 0.2 to 0.5 mm in diameter were observed on the 5th day after inoculation and attained sizes of 1.0 to 2.0 mm by day 11. However, microscopic observation revealed numerous microplaques which could not be counted macroscopically, accounting for the fact that tube infectivity titers exceeded those obtained in the plaque assay by 10^1 to $10^{1.5}$ $TCID_{50}$.

Harrison et al. (1968) showed plaque formation in BS-C-1 cells, a diploid cell line derived from African green monkey kidney cells. Distemper virus, that had been adapted to BS-C-1 cells, was inoculated into monolayers. The virus was allowed to adsorb for 1 hour at room temperature and the plates were then overlaid with agar medium. Plate cultures were reincubated at 37° C in 5 per cent CO_2. Plaque counts 14 days later showed a linear relation with the inoculated virus dose. When plaque counts were made after 9 or 12 days, the average was only 39 or 86 per cent of the 14 day results.

A plaque system with the Lederle strain of CDV in Vero cells, a carboxymethyl cellulose overlay and a 10 day incubation period was used by Gourlay (1970).

7. Fluorescent Antibody Labelling

Although the fluorescent antibody (FA) method is commonly used for the detection of CD viral antigen in cells, only one sequential study has been published (Yamanouchi et al., 1970). They used the Vero cell-adapted Lederle strain of CDV in Vero cells with a multiplicity of infection of 0.1. The direct FA technique was employed. At 12 hours PI, few fluorescent granules were demonstrated in the cytoplasms around the nuclear membrane. Size and number of granules increased with time. At 24 hours PI fluorescence filled the cytoplasms and increased in intensity up to 48 hours. Intranuclear fluorescence appeared only 48 to 72 hours PI, together with the first giant cell formation. Intensely fluorescing areas corresponded with inclusion bodies. However, inclusion bodies tend to persist longer than fluorescing granules (v. Mickwitz and Schröder, 1968). In several day old giant cells, massive inclusions can be stained but fluorescence becomes very faint.

8. Indirect Hemadsorption

An indirect hemadsorption was observed in CDV infected cell cultures (Fagraeus and Espmark, 1961). Infected cells were first incubated with CDV antiserum prepared in rabbits. After 1 hour, cell cultures were washed several times to remove unbound serum. Sheep red blood cells coated with horse-anti-rabbit serum was then added and hemadsorption was seen around infected foci.

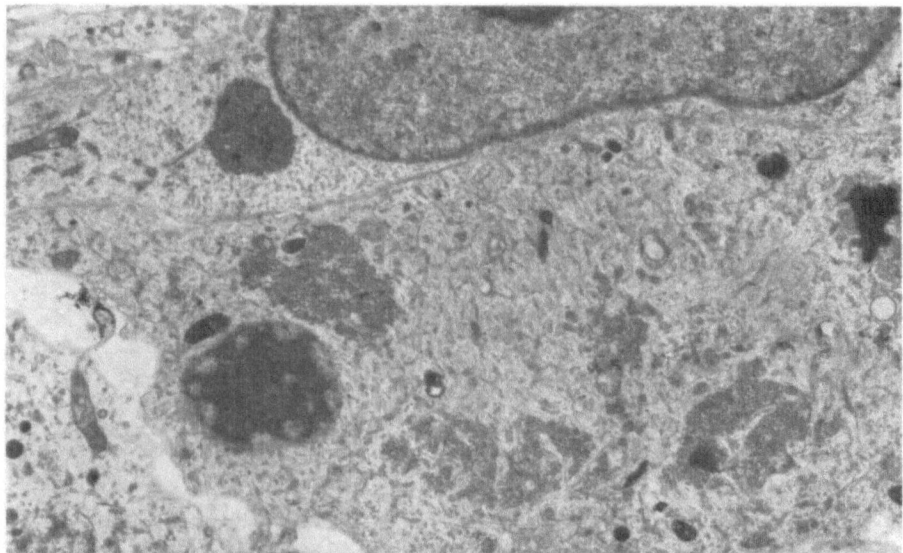

Fig. 10. CDV-infected cerebellar explant (14th p. i. d.). Astrocyte with several intracytoplasmic tubular aggregates. Notice glial filaments (× 11,250). Reprinted with permission from: KOESTNER, A. and J., LONG, Lab. Invest. **23,** 196 (1970)

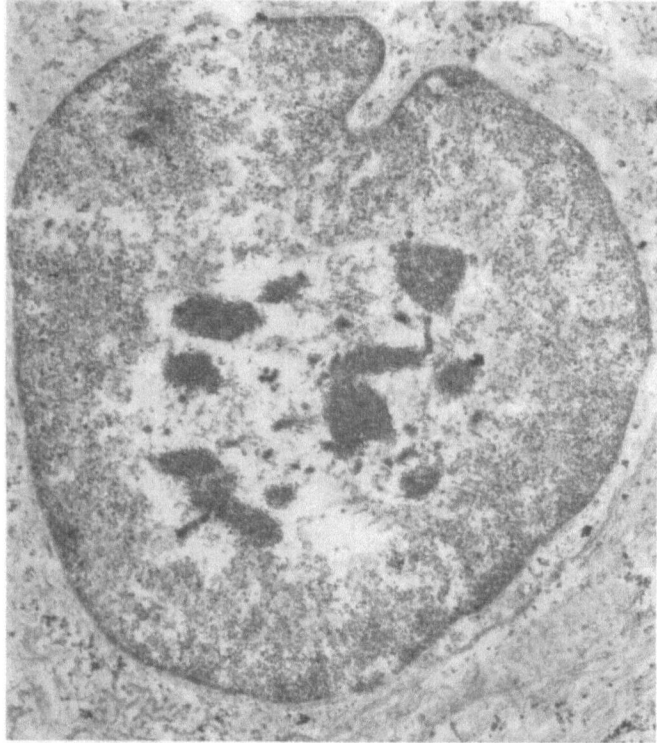

Fig. 11. CDV-infected cerebellar explant (23rd p. i. d.). Intranuclear viral capsids in crystalline arrangement (× 18,300). Reprinted with permission from: KOESTNER, A. and J. LONG: Lab. Invest. **23,** 196 (1970)

9. Electron Microscopy

Sequential studies of CDV cell infection by electron microscopy have been made by KOESTNER and LONG (1970). They infected canine cerebellar explant cultures with the Lederle strain. Viral capsids (Fig. 10) were first demonstrated in the cytoplasm of glial cells and macrophages on the 7th day PI coinciding with the appearance of inclusion bodies detectable by light microscopy. Between 2 and

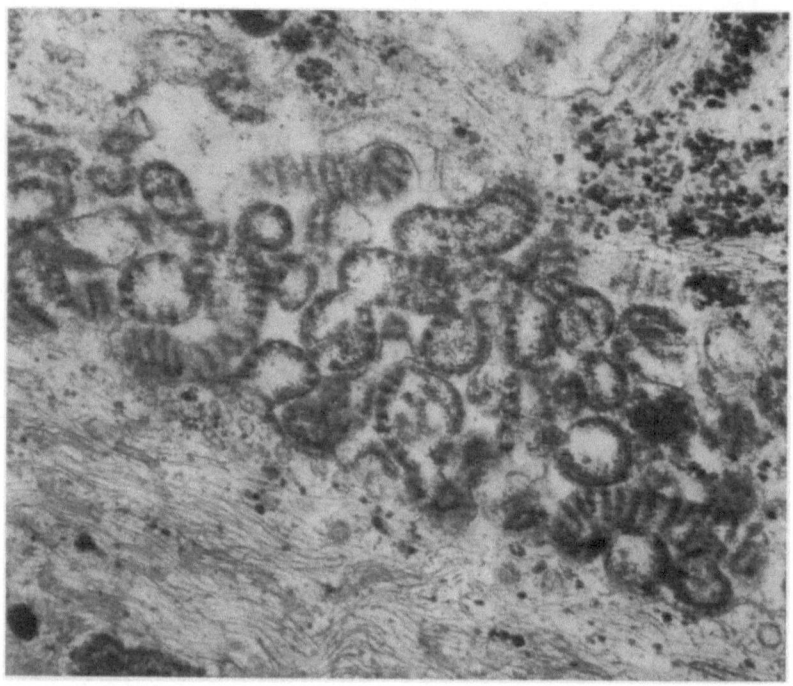

Fig. 12. CDV-infected cerebellar explant (23rd p. i. d.). Membrane of astrocytic process is lined by viral capsids. Notice glial filaments (× 38,300). Reprinted with permission from: KOESTNER, A. and J. LONG: Lab. Invest. **23**, 196 (1970)

3 weeks following infection viral capsids also appeared in nuclei (Fig. 11) where they were mostly arranged in crystalline arrays, coinciding with the occurrence of intranuclear inclusion bodies. Viral nucleocapsids lined cellular membranes and virus particles were formed by budding (Fig. 12). Similar results were obtained by TAJIMA et al. (1971). Cytoplasmic and intranuclear inclusions in CDV infected CEF and Vero cells were composed of viral nucleocapsids which were enveloped by budding at the cell surface.

IV. Interaction with Organisms

A. Pathogenesis

1. Natural Host Range

Canine distemper virus (CDV) has a wide host range in animal populations. Animals of the order *Carnivora*, suborder *Fissepeda* or land carnivores are affected. All animals in the *Canidae*, *Procyonidae* and *Mustelidae* families seem to be susceptible although proof is lacking for some species. Carnivores of the *Hyaenidae* and *Ursidae* families appear to be resistant. The *Viverridae* family is probably resistant but there is one report of distemper in a Binturong (Goss, 1948). *Felidae* were thought to be resistant. However, domestic cats develop an inapparent and abortive infection after experimental exposure to CDV (cf. p. 33). Inapparent CDV infections probably occur in more families. The pathogenicity of CDV varies from species to species from inapparent infection to a 100 per cent mortality.

Goss (1948) tabulated the distemper susceptible species. Gorham (1960 and 1966) referred to this table summarizing the host range. v. Mickwitz (1968) recommended a change, because he diagnosed distemper in animals of the *Procyonidae* group other than the raccoon. The altered table is presented here (Table 3).

Three criteria were generally accepted to confirm the diagnosis of canine distemper, before virus isolation in tissue culture and the fluorescent antibody method became known: (1) Inclusion bodies, predominately intracytoplasmic, some intra-

Table 3. *Natural Host Range of Canine Distemper*[1]

Order Carnivora:

  Suborder Fissipeda: terrestrial Carnivora

Family Felidae:	cats, *lions*, tigers, etc. (questionable)
Family Viverridae:	civets, fossa, mongoose, meerkat, linsang, *binturong* (questionable)
Family Hyaenidae:	hyenas
Family Canidae:	*dogs, dingo, fox, coyote, wolf, jackal* (all susceptible)
Family Procyonidae:	*kinkajou, coati, bassariscus, raccoon, panda* (probably all susceptible)
Family Mustelidae:	*weasel, ferret, mink, skunk, badger, stoat, marten, otter* (all susceptible)
Family Ursidae:	bears

---

[1] Reported species in italics.

nuclear in various tissues; (2) virus transmission and production of the disease in ferrets and dogs; and (3) complement fixation of tissue suspensions from infected animals with specific antiserum. Reports from the early part of this century were based on clinical observations and are not considered to be specific (McGowan, 1911; Fox, 1923; Schröder, 1925).

One of the first species besides dogs known to be susceptible to CDV was the domestic ferret *(Mustela putorius)*. Dunkin and Laidlaw (1926 a) used it extensively for their studies with distemper. They mentioned that distemper in ferrets trained for rabbit hunting had been known for a long time. Since the mortality rate in ferrets is nearly 100 per cent, this animal was commonly used for virus transmission and titration studies until recently (Crook et al., 1958).

Distemper in the silver fox *(Vulpes vulpes)* was first demonstrated by Green (1926). He filtered blood serum from distemper-diseased foxes through Berkefeld N filters and produced the disease with filtrates. Rudolf (1930) reported distemper in silver fox, mink, and raccoon. Dedie et al. (1957) reviewed the literature and described distemper in the silver fox. The clinical picture was often less severe than in dogs, but complications with *Salmonella* organism were common. The mortality in adults was 20 per cent and in cubs 80 per cent.

SHAW (1933) described outbreaks of canine distemper on mink farms. He stated that the disease was widespread in the United States and Canada. Adult mink *(Mustela vison)* showed a considerable resistance to the disease while kits were almost 100 per cent susceptible. He based his diagnosis on clinical observations, negative bacteriological examination, and no gross pathologic lesions. Numerous reports on distemper in mink followed from Europe and America (PINKERTON, 1940; MOMBERG-JÖRGENSEN, 1949; GORHAM, 1952; DE HAAN, 1954; SCHINDLER, 1955). BINDRICH et al. (1959) gave a review with a detailed description of canine distemper in mink. They based the diagnosis of CD on the presence of inclusion bodies in various tissues and on a positive complement-fixation test. They found the disease to be very common in mink. Mortality was found to be between 40 and 60 per cent. Two forms of the disease were observed: One resulting in sudden death, the other was more chronic with catarrhal signs followed by nervous manifestations.

MARTINAGLIA (1937) described an outbreak among silver jackals *(Vulpes chama)* in the menagerie of the Johannesburg, South Africa, zoo. HAMERTON (1937) reported an epizootic described as canine distemper among *Canidae* in a London zoo. The following species were affected: the jackal *(Canis adustus)*, the Karagan fox *(Vulpes karagan)*, the dingo *(Canis dingo)*, and the wolf *(Lupus* sp.).

ARMSTRONG and ANTHONY (1942) observed an epizootic in an exhibition unit of *Canidae* and *Felidae*. All the *Canidae* but none of the *Felidae* showed signs of the disease. The *Canidae* included: red foxes *(Vulpus fulva)*, gray foxes *(Urocyon cinereoargenteus)*, kit foxes *(Vulpus macrotis)*, South American foxes *(Dusicyon* sp.), Australian dingoes *(Canis dingo)*, raccoon dogs *(Canis procyonoides)*, Eurasian badger *(Meles meles)*, and coyote-dog hybrids. A spleen suspension from a gray fox was inoculated into a ferret, the ferret died 14 days later with symptoms of acute distemper. Inclusion bodies were seen in smear preparations from urinary bladders and tissue sections. They were reported to be relatively small and mostly intranuclear. Cytoplasmic inclusion bodies were uncommon.

Later in the same year, ARMSTRONG (1942) inoculated spleen suspensions from distemper-infected ferrets subcutaneously into 4 American badgers *(Taxidea taxus)*. The animals developed distemper symptoms and died between 12 and 18 days postinoculation. The susceptibility of this species was confirmed by GORHAM (1966); a badger died from distemper 15 days after an unusual route of exposure (Discussion to GORHAM, 1966). FISCHER (1965) found distemper inclusion bodies in glial cells of 4 Eurasian badgers *(Meles meles)*. The animals had been rabies suspects.

Additional species of the *Mustelidae* family susceptible to CD have been discussed and reported by KEYMER and EPPS (1969). They found CD in the stoat *(Mustela erminea)*, the weasel *(M. nivalis)* and the least weasel *(M. rixosa)*. They presumed the CD susceptible "Wiesel" reported by BINDRICH (1962) to be *M. nivalis* and the "Marder" to be a *Mustela* species of marten, and the "otter" reported by FISCHER (1965) to be a *Lutra* species. SEDGWICK and YOUNG (1968) reported CD in the Allamand's grison *(Galictis vittata)*.

HELMBOLDT and JUNGHERR (1955) pointed to the importance of differential diagnosis between rabies and distemper in wild living carnivores. They found distemper in gray foxes, red foxes, raccoons, and skunks *(Mephitis mephitis)*, which had shown signs similar to those of rabies. Negri bodies could not be found in the brain, and mouse-inoculation tests were negative, but typical distemper inclusion bodies were found in various tissues. Ferrets died from distemper when inoculated with brain material. Similar findings were made by ROBINSON et al. (1957) and HABERMANN et al. (1958). PARKER et al. (1961) found distemper antibodies in foxes and raccoons, but not in the opossum.

KILHAM et al. (1954, 1956) found distemper in raccoons and ferrets producing bilirubinaemia and jaundice. KARSTADT and BUDD (1964) described 9 cases of distemper in wild raccoons with a giant cell type pneumonitis. CROOK and McNUTT (1958) passaged distemper virus from a raccoon to a ferret and adapted it to embryonated hens' eggs. GRÜNBERG (1959) found distemper in 2 huskies and 4 dingoes in a zoo.

SEDGWICK and YOUNG (1968) described a CD outbreak in a zoo, including North American and maned wolves, raccoon dogs, South American fox dogs, and badgers.

Recently (v. MICKWITZ, 1968), the letter panda has been included in the group of distemper-susceptible animals. He considered all animals in the Procyonides-group to be susceptible to CD. The diagnosis was made in 8 letter pandas and in one kinkajou. Distemper-like signs were seen. Four of the eight animals had salmonellosis besides distemper infection. Principally cytoplasmic, but also some intranuclear inclusion bodies were found in many tissues and cells. Viral antigen was seen with fluorescent antibody (v. MICKWITZ and SCHRÖDER, 1967). Feulgen and PAS staining of inclusion bodies was negative. An earlier report (ANONYM., 1960) described canine distemper in pandas in the Cheyenne Mountain zoo and in the London zoo. Transmission to ferrets induced distemper. The disease occurred most often in recently imported pandas. MÜLLER (1962) made note of distemper in a coati.

Goss (1948) included the binturong in the distemper-susceptible group. He described one outbreak in these animals, which died with distemper signs of illness. No attempt was made to transmit the virus to other animals. Intranuclear and cytoplasmic inclusions were seen and one figure with intranuclear inclusions in cells of kidney tubules was shown. OTT and CABASSO (discussion to GORHAM, 1966) questioned the specificity of the inclusion bodies. Until confirmed, the susceptibility of the binturong to distemper remains doubtful.

PIAT (1950) observed distemper in two 4-month-old lion cubs which came in contact with a one-year-old Cocker Spaniel. Infection of their blood into two susceptible dogs caused distemper signs. Because the *Felidae* family was not considered susceptible to CDV, this report was taken with caution. However, cats were recently found to be susceptible to CDV, producing inapparent infections (APPEL et al., 1971). Susceptibility of wild animal species to CD should be further investigated.

2. Experimental Host Range

a) Embryonated Chicken Eggs

After GOODPASTURE and WOODRUFF (1931) had demonstrated that several viruses could be propagated on the chorioallantoic membrane (CAM) of embryonating chicken eggs, and after BURNET (1937) had shown that numerous passages through embryonated eggs rendered influenza virus avirulent for mice and ferrets, numerous attempts were made to adapt distemper virus to embryonating eggs.

MITSCHERLICH (1938) inoculated blood, taken at the time of the first temperature peak from distemper infected dogs, on the CAM of 9-day-old embryonated hen's eggs. After incubation for 3 days at 38° C, a piece of the CAM was transferred to the CAM of other embryonated eggs. Three days later a whitish thickening on the membrane was observed and a suspension of these infected membranes produced distemper in a dog. Further CDV passages in eggs were unsuccessful.

HAIG (1948) was the first to maintain distemper virus in serial passages in eggs. The strain developed by him was designated the "Onderstepoort" strain. It lost its contagiousness for ferrets after 25 passages (HAIG, 1956). HAIG began with a spleen suspension of a ferret which had been inoculated with ferret-adapted distemper virus (GREEN, 1939) in the 57th passage. Eight-day embryonated eggs were inoculated on the CAM and incubated at 35° C. A passage was made after 4 days, when a slight thickening of the membranes was observed. Passages in eggs were carried aut 30 times. A marked thickening of the membranes and gray foci were noted after 9 passages. Later (1956), HAIG found the 130th passage to be safe for use as vaccine for both dogs and ferrets.

CABASSO and COX (1949) soon afterwards reported similar results. Their egg-adapted CDV strain was designated "Lederle" and it lost its virulence for ferrets between the 24th and 28th passage. This strain has been widely used vor vaccination of CD susceptible animals.

The adaptation of distemper virus to eggs has been repeated in several laboratories (LUCAM and GORET, 1951; CABASSO and COX, 1952; LASFARGUES, 1953; BINDRICH, 1954; MANTOVANI, 1954; WEST et al., 1956; CROOK and MCNUTT, 1958) using different strains of virus for primary inoculations. Optimal results were obtained with 7-day-old embryonating chicken eggs for inoculations, incubation at 37° C and harvesting membranes 6 to 7 days later (GORHAM, 1957 a).

GORHAM (1960) mentioned the passage of chicken egg-adapted virus to embryonated duck eggs. Lesions on CAMs of duck eggs were as prominent as on chicken egg membranes.

STÜNZI et al. (1954) studied the pathological response of the CAM to adapted distemper virus. They used the Onderstepoort and the Lederle strains of virus in their experiments in 7-day-old chicken embryos maintained at 37° C. They found hyperplasia of the epithelium on day one PI. In addition, edema and proliferation of mesenchymal cells were seen 2 days PI. A few epithelial cells showed pyknosis and karyorrhexis. After 5 days the inflammatory reaction was more evident, with leukocyte infiltration. Mitoses in mesenchymal and epithelial cells were numerous. After 7 days some blood vessels showed thrombosis and endangitis. From 7 to 12 days the inflammatory reaction diminished. Thrombosed arterioles and areas of abundant granulocytes were seen in some infected membranes. Virus titration of infected membranes in eggs showed greatest concentration of virus and the peak of inflammatory reactions. WEST et al. (1956) and CROOK (1957) reported similar results. WEST et al. (1956) found acidophilic intracytoplasmic inclusion bodies in ectodermal cells. BELCHER (1951) and MONTOVANI (1954 a) also reported acidophilic inclusions. CROOK (1957) pointed out that inclusions were not observed in membranes inoculated with the raccoon 9, Wisconsin FXNO, and Lederle variants. Continued passage resulted in a reversion of plaque-forming capability to a more pronounced thickening and edema of the CAMs (GORHAM, 1960).

Electron microscopy of CDV replication in CAMs has been reported by LAWN (1970).

The effect of CDV on the developing chick embryo in infected eggs has not been studied. Chicks from CDV infected eggs hatch without feathers.

b) Mice

In an attempt to produce vaccine strains of canine distemper, MANSEY (1948) inoculated mice intracerebrally with the virulent Cairo and Wellcome strains. In a later discussion (MACINTYRE et al., 1948) he reported nervous symptoms and deaths of these mice 6 to 8 days after inoculation. The different strains had different incubation periods. No attempt was mentioned to identify the virus after passage in mice, and the specificity was questioned.

KLAPÖTKE (1953) inoculated adult white mice intracerebrally with virulent distemper spleen suspensions. Virus could be passaged from mouse brain to dogs 4 days after inoculation. Attempts to transfer this virus to mouse brain were not successful. However, distemper virus that was propagated in mouse embryo brain explants for 18 passages did adapt to adult white mouse brains. Twelve mouse-brain passages were made with this virus.

BINDRICH (1954) inoculated dog brain suspension with virulent CDV (Greifswald strain) in the 65th passage into the cerebral hemispheres of adult white mice and passaged brain in 3-days intervals. Although the mice did not show any signs, distemper virus was still present after 14 brain passages and dogs given this passage became infected with typical signs of CD.

MORSE et al. (1953) adapted and maintained CDV in mouse-brain passages. Beginning with the egg-adapted "FXNO" strain, which originated from an infected fox spleen, they inoculated CAM suspensions of the 65th and 75th passages into the cerebral hemispheres of 1-to-4-day-old Swiss albino mice. From the first to the tenth passage the incubation period was reduced from 8 to 3 days with brain virus titers in moribund mice increasing correspondingly. In early passages the most striking symptoms occurring were running and jumping in cages for 2 to 3 days, before mice were euthanized. After the eight passage, incoordination, ataxia, clonic spasms, and paresis were more prominent. The immunizing effect of this mouse-brain-adapted strain was demonstrated in ferrets, and neutralization tests in mice were performed to identify the virus. When infected-mouse-brain suspensions were inoculated into embryonated eggs, three or four passages in eggs were required to produce characteristic lesions.

The adaptation of avianized CDV to suckling mice with similar results was repeated frequently (GUTIEREZ and GORHAM, 1955; CARLSTRÖM, 1956; ADAMS and IMAGAWA, 1957; IMAGAWA and ADAMS, 1958; ARAKAWA et al., 1959; and FUJIE, 1964). CABASSO et al. (1955) succeeded after serial CDV passage in suckling hamster brain.

WEST and BRANDLY (1955) reported the adaptation of virulent fox distemper virus to mouse lungs. Three-week-old white mice were inoculated intranasally under light ether anesthesia with spleen, lymph node, and lung suspensions of two distemper strains which were fatal for fox pups within 3 to 5 days. The inoculation was repeated 24 hours later, mice were euthanized 48 hours after the last inoculation. This procedure was repeated throughout 40 passages using mouse lung suspensions as inoculum. In the first passage, 50 per cent of infected mice had consolidated areas in the lungs. The percentage increased with subsequent passages. The effect was neutralized with distemper immune serum from foxes, but not with normal fox serum. Foxes inoculated with the 25th mouse passage lung material developed distemper signs. Contact transmission from mouse to mouse did not occur. Adult mice were refractory to intracerebral or intraperitoneal inoculation with the mouse-propagated material. Attempts to repeat the adaptation with less virulent fox strains of CDV failed. Since a fatal effect from distemper virus alone in fox pups within 3 to 5 days is unusual, the question arises whether a second agent was present in the original material.

c) Hamsters

CABASSO et al. (1955) adapted the 44th passage of the Lederle strain to brains of hamsters 3 to 5 days of age. Seven days after the initial inoculation some animals were found dead. The survivors showed apathy, incoordination, slow movements, and rolling on their backs when disturbed. Serial passages were performed which reduced the incubation period from the initial 7 days to 4 days after 16 passages. Signs remained unchanged. When inoculated into embryonated eggs, the hamster-propagated virus produced typical distemper lesions on CAMs. Serum-neutralization tests were made successfully in suckling hamsters. The immunization effect of infected hamster brain was shown in ferrets. Mouse-adapted CDV was adapted to suckling hamster with similar results (GUITEREZ and GORHAM, 1955).

MOTOHASHI et al. (1964) adapted an egg-propagated strain of CD virus to suckling hamster brain. Once adapted, weanling and adult hamsters became susceptible by intracerebral, but not by peritoneal or intranasal inoculation. Nervous signs appeared 4 to 7 days postinoculation and mortality rate was 100 per cent after 10 passages.

ARMSTRONG and BURNSTEIN (1966) adapted attenuated CDV to suckling and older hamsters and described clinical signs and histopathological lesions. Suckling hamsters had incoordination, opisthotonus, stunting, dehydration, and death. Meningitis and necrosis of the olfactory bulbs, cerebrum, and ependyma were seen. Signs of illness in weanling and adult hamsters were ptyalism, convulsions and death. Brain edema, neuronal degeneration, mononuclear cell infiltration of vessel walls and meningitis were described. Demyelination and inclusion bodies were not seen.

d) Rabbits

GORET et al. (1952) inoculated rabbits subcutaneously with virulent distemper ferret brain suspensions. They repeated the inoculation 48 hours later. Using rabbit spleen suspensions for passages, the double exposure was repeated 25 times. After six passages the authors found a raised temperature response in 80 to 100 per cent of infected rabbits. After 7 to 9 passages the virus lost its virulence for ferrets. It also had no immunizing capacity and inoculated ferrets did not respond with antibody formation. Distemper virus, therefore, was probably not present.

MARTIN (1950) claimed distemper virus adaptation to the rabbit with temperature rise and spleen enlargements seen in rabbits. Virus identity was not shown.

LÜHRS (1926), using different routes of inoculation in 200 rabbits, KANTORO-WICZ (1933), attempting virus transmission in 155 rabbits, and BINDRICH (1954) came to the conclusion that distemper virus could not be adapted to rabbits. BINDRICH attempted intravenous, intracerebral, and intraperitoneal inoculations with serial rabbit and alternating rabbit-dog passages. Intranasal infection with virulent CDV did not produce infection in rabbits (APPEL, unpublished).

e) Rats

Several transmission attempts of distemper virus to white rats were reported to be unsuccessful (LAIDLAW and DUNKIN, 1926; KANTOROWICZ, 1933; BINDRICH, 1954).

f) Cats

Cat distemper, a parvovirus infection, was earlier confused with canine distemper (SCHRÖDER, 1925). However, domestic cats were recently found to be susceptible to CDV (APPEL et al., unpublished). Newborn, 6-week-old, and adult cats were inoculated intranasally with spleen suspensions from CDV (Snyder Hill strain) infected SPF dogs. Cats did not produce clinical disease and virus did not spread from cats to dogs but CDV was isolated in dog lung macrophages (APPEL and JONES, 1967) from lymphatic tissues of infected cats 5 and 6 days PI. Serial passages in cats were made and virus titers did not decrease with passages. Foci of infected cells in lymphatic tissues were seen with fluorescent antibody. A significant reduction in size of the thymus in newborn cats 5 to 6 days PI was the only gross lesion observed. Histopathological changes included interlobular edema in the thymus with proteinaceous exudation, and degeneration and a marked reduction of lymphocytes within the lobules. Neutralizing antibody was found in cat serum 7 days PI and virus could not be isolated at that time. There was no virus spread to epithelial cells or brain like in dogs (cf. p. 37). The CDV passaged in cats was not related to the cat syncytial virus (GASKIN, unpublished).

g) Pigs

Similar to the domestic cat, Yorkshire pigs and African minipigs were recently found to be susceptible to CDV (APPEL et al., unpublished). Newborn and weaned Yorkshire piglets and 2-year-old minipigs were inoculated intranasally with spleen suspension from CDV (Snyder Hill strain) infected SPF dogs. Newborn piglets developed bronchopneumonia with secondary bacterial infection not observed in control littermates. Weaned and adult pigs remained without clinical signs. Virus did not spread from pig to pig. Virus isolation, serial passages, and pathology were very similar to those in cats. Focal splenic necroses both within the sinusoidal region and within splenic corpuscles was seen in some pigs. Virus replication, like in cats, was restricted to lymphatic tissues and virus could not be isolated 7 days PI or more, when neutralizing antibody appeared in pig serum.

h) Monkeys

Neutralizing antibody to CDV was found in monkeys after MV infection (see Immunological Relationship between CDV and MV, p. 48). MARTIN (1950) reported encephalitis and death in the Macaca sylvanus inoculated with CDV. However, the syndrome in monkeys was not differentiated from infection with human poliomyelitis virus and monkeys immune to the latter did not develop clinical signs with CDV.

DELAY et al. (1965) found a transitory febrile reaction in young cynomolgous monkeys for 10 days after subcutaneous inoculation with virulent (Snyder Hill) CDV.

i) Man

NICOLLE (1931) inoculated human volunteers with CDV. It produced an inapparent infection with a viremia for at least 6 days, detected by blood inoculation into susceptible dogs.

3. Development of Virus in the Host

Although ferrets, mink, or dogs can be experimentally infected with distemper virus by any route, the natural route of infection appears to be aerosol and droplet exposure. LAIDLAW and DUNKIN (1926a) demonstrated the air transmission in ferrets by placing susceptible animals in cages several feet away from exposed animals. Ten days later the unexposed ferrets developed signs of distemper. Therefore, the authors used the pavilion arrangement of kennels, where each animal unit was 15 to 20 meters apart from the neighboring unit. Because distemper in ferrets and dogs is highly contagious, the concept of air transmission has not been questioned since.

The spread and development of CDV in the host has only been studied in ferrets, mink, and dogs which will be discussed in more detail. It must be assumed that the initial infection is the same in all susceptible species after aerosol or droplet exposure. Virus replication occurs first in local macrophages which transport the virus to lymphatic tissues. Virus spreads to spleen, thymus, and bone marrow within a few days. If neutralizing antibody appears within one week PI the infection remains inapparent and virus can no longer be isolated from suspended tissues. If animals fail to produce protective levels of neutralizing antibody within the second week PI, virus spreads to epithelium of many organs and to the brain, resulting in clinical disease with a high mortality rate.

a) In Ferrets and Mink

LIU and COFFIN (1957) used the immunofluorescence technique to follow the site of entry and spread of virus in ferrets after intranasal inoculation with virulent virus. They exposed a total of 21 ferrets 4 to 15 months old, euthanized them in various intervals and took various tissue samples or smear preparations from each animal.

The clinical course of distemper in these experimentally infected ferrets was similar to that described by DUNKIN and LAIDLAW (1926a). The onset of fever varied from the 4th to the 6th day post-inoculation, erythematous cutaneous lesions appeared one to 4 days thereafter. After the onset of fever, most ferrets were inactive and anoretic. Later, erythema and swelling of anus, eye, and eyelids appeared. Purulent conjunctivitis was common. Loss of weight was prominent and ferrets became moribund within 4 to 5 days after the onset of fever. Between time of exposure and death of ferrets, the following spread and distribution of viral antigen in tissues was found: On the 2nd day post-infection (PI) viral antigen was seen in the cytoplasm of a few reticular cells of the cervical lymph node medullary sinuses. On the 3rd and 4th day, most of the cells in the same lymph nodes contained antigen and the lymphoid follicles were packed with fluorescent lymphocytes. At the same time viral antigen appeared in mediastinal and mesenteric lymph nodes, in splenic white pulp, and in some reticular cells in red pulp of the spleen. It also was found in leukocytes of peripheral blood in smear preparations, predominately in the cytoplasm of mononuclear cells. By the 6th and 7th day, almost all cells in the lymph nodes examined and in the spleen showed intracytoplasmic fluorescence. The tonsil, lymphocytes, and the covering squamous epithelium contained antigen. In the gastrointestinal tract, viral antigen was seen in lymphoid nodules along the basement membrane and in lymphocytes in the lamina propria of stomach, duodenum, and ileum mucosa. Kupffer cells in the liver and bile duct epithelial cells showed fluorescence as well as some pancreatic duct and acinar cells. Nine and 10 days PI a general spread to epithelial cells was noted. In the respiratory tract, tracheal and bronchial epithelium had cytoplasmic fluorescent granules ranging from fine granules to large oval bodies. Many cells in the alveolar septa and peribronchial tissues contained viral antigen. In the gastrointestinal tract, viral antigen was seen in cells of the gastric glands but seldom in epithelium of the small intestine. In the urinary tract it appeared in the cytoplasm of renal pelvic epithelium and bladder epithelium. In cutaneous tissue viral antigen was seen in the epithelium of hair follicles, in sebacious and sweat glands, and in focal distribution in the epidermis. Conjunctival swab preparations were positive. Only two ferrets survived 14 and 15 days and viral antigen was only seen in vascular endothelial cells of the brain.

In H and E stained paraffin sections, distemper inclusion bodies were found where viral antigen labelled with fluorescent antibody was most abundant. A striking hyper- and parakeratosis of epidermis including footpads, hair follicles, and sebacious glands was noted.

In contrast to the concept of LIU and COFFIN (1957) who demonstrated reticuloendothelial and lymphatic tissue to be site of entry for distemper virus, CROOK et al. (1958) and CROOK and McNUTT (1959) considered nasal mucosa and lung to be the site of initial virus replication. CROOK et al. (1958) used lung and spleen suspensions from ferrets infected with Green's distemperoid virus strain to expose 10-to-20-week old ferrets and mink by aerosol. Two animals each were euthanized on consecutive days and various tissue suspensions were titrated in susceptible ferrets to determine virus concentration. In ferrets, virus was present in nasal tissues, lung, spleen, and blood 2 days after aerosol exposure. From 3 to 6 days a steady virus increase was found in nasal tissue, lung, and spleen with little increase thereafter. Virus concentration in the blood remained lower and fairly constant. Virus also appeared in liver and brain 3 days after exposure. Virus was present in nasal tissues and lung on the 2nd day PI. It appeared in the blood on the 3rd day, and the kidney, bladder, brain, liver, and muscle one day later. The increase in nasal tissues was observed again, although it was slower than in ferrets. Increases in kidney, bladder, brain, and liver were also noticed. In some animals that had been infected 16 days or more, virus was also found in adrenal, salivary, and thyroid glands.

A fairly high virus titer was present early in the blood and consequently in all organs. Because the lung contains peribronchial lymphatic tissue, the evaluation of entry of CDV into the host was difficult. The histopathology of these species was described by CROOK and McNUTT (1959). The first lesions were found on the 4th day of infection and included necrosis of the spleen.

b) In Dogs

The natural route of distemper infection in dogs, as in ferrets, is by air and droplet exposure. Distemper in dogs differs considerably from the disease in ferrets. The mortality rate in ferrets is almost 100 per cent, in dogs it is approximately 50 per cent. Ferrets usually do not produce protective antibody levels against CDV when exposed to virulent virus. The outcome of the disease in dogs depended on the capacity of individual dogs to form antibody (OTT et al., 1955; ROCKBORN 1957; FAIRCHILD, 1967; APPEL, 1969).

CARRÉ (1905) demonstrated viremia in distemper in dogs. Passaging blood from dog to dog during the first febrile period, he found blood to contain virus 3 to 6 days after inoculation. LAIDLAW and DUNKIN (1926 a, 1928 a) confirmed CARRÉ's observation. Sequential events in dogs were first studied by BINDRICH (1950 a, b, 1954). He found viremia first at the time of the first temperature peak; viremia lasted in one dog for 41 days. BINDRICH thought distemper virus was attached to erythrocytes, because repeated washings eliminated virus. The washing probably also eliminated leukocytes which are known to contain virus (LIU and COFFIN, 1957). BINDRICH found that virus spread to various organs several days after viremia had occurred. Titrating virus in dogs, he found highest virus titers in spleen, mesenteric lymph nodes, bone marrow, kidney, and brain. After virus inoculation into cerebrospinal fluid, a similar sequence of events occurred as a viremia was followed by spreads to various organs including brain.

ROCKBORN (1957, 1958) found an inverse relationship between presence of virus and antibody. He inoculated pups with a virulent Swedish strain and found viremia 4 and 6, but not 8 and 10 days after intramuscular injection. The virus was found in the cellular fraction but not in the plasma. Antibody levels were 1 : 30 or less on day 6; they increased to 1 : 100 or greater on day 10. OTT (1955) also had noticed low antibody titers in dogs with fatal distemper.

COFFIN and LIU (1957) studied the distribution of viral antigen with fluorescent antibody in three groups of dogs with distemper infection; (1) acute systemic infection; (2) combined systemic and central nervous system (CNS) infection; (3) chiefly CNS infection. In the first group, viral antigen was found in cells of the lymphatic system and in epithelial cells of many organs but not in brain cells. In the second group, it had spread to glial cells, ependymal cells and neurons in the brain. In the third group, virus was predominantly seen in cells in the brain. The three groups of infected dogs probably represented three different phases in relation to antibody formation. Similar results were reported by v. MICKWITZ and SCHRÖDER (1968) (see: Diagnosis, p. 68).

CORNWELL et al. (1965) exposed dogs by contact to virulent distemper virus from street cases. They found a diphasic viremia in dogs, the first phase occurring between 5 and 8 days ,the second, which was found only in severe cases, beginning 3 to 10 days later, and lasting until death. Virus isolation was made in ferret kidney cells (VANTSIS, 1959). The diphasic viremia was related to a diphasic temperature response. Virus persisted in the lung and spinal cord of one dog 57 days post-inoculation, which was 4 weeks after virus was present in the blood. The nonsynchronous elimination of virus from different organs was also reported by LAUDER *et al.* (1954) and COFFIN and LIU (1957).

APPEL (1969) exposed specific pathogen-free Beagle dogs to virulent CDV by aerosol in a Middlebrook chamber (MIDDLEBROOK, 1952). Frozen tissue sections from 64 dogs were examined during the course of the disease, using the direct fluorescent antibody method for detection of viral antigen (Table 4). Course of the disease and presence of viral antigen in different organs were related to presence of serum-neutralizing antibody. Two days PI, viral antigen was found in a few mononuclear cells situated in the sinus of bronchial lymph nodes and tonsils. During the first week PI, virus spread rapidly in blood leukocytes; cells in spleen (Fig. 13), thymus, bone marrow, various lymph nodes, lamina propria of stomach and intestine, and Kupffer cells in liver had viral antigen but not epithelial cells or brain cells. Between 6 and 9 days mononuclear cells in connective tissue of various organs contained viral antigen and only single epithelial cells (Fig. 14). First neutralizing (SN) antibody in serum was found after 8 or 9 days. Approximately 50 per cent of dogs produced antibody rapidly. Viral antigen was not seen in these dogs 2 and 3 weeks PI and they did not develop clinical signs, with few exceptions. The other 50 per cent of the dogs failed to produce protective antibody levels. Viral antigen in these dogs became widespread and was present in surface epithelium of alimentary (Fig. 15), respiratory, urogenital tracts, and in exocrine and endocrine glands in addition to the earlier distribution. In the brain, first viral antigen appear-

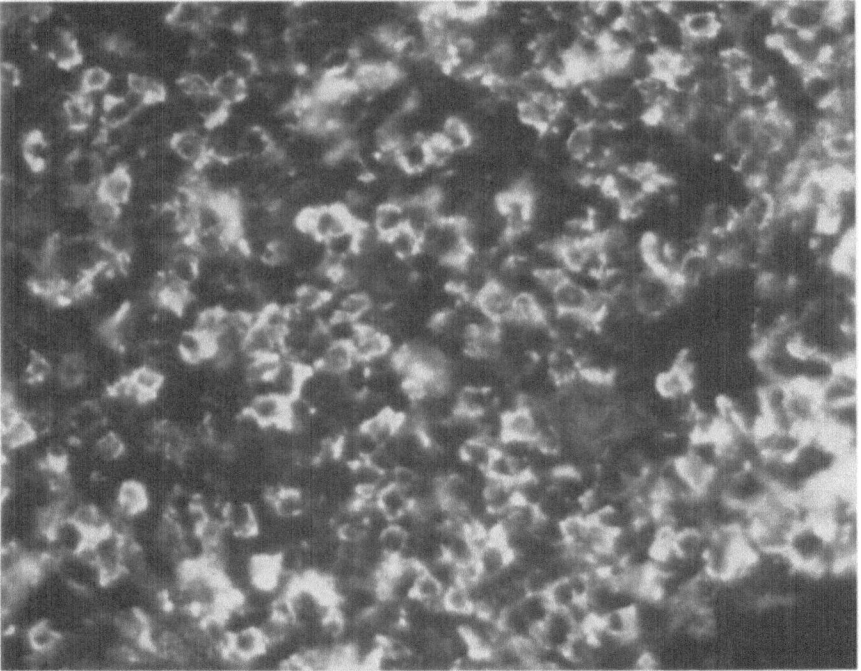

Fig. 13. Extensive, predominately intracytoplasmic fluorescence in spleen of dog 7 days after it was exposed to aerosol of canine distemper virus (× 250). Reprinted with permission from: APPEL, M. J. G.: Amer. J. vet. Res. **30**, 1167 (1969)

Table 4. *Distribution of Canine Distemper Virus Given in the Form of Aerosol to 64 Dogs*

| | | | | | Days after exposure | | | | |
| | | | | | 14—16 | | 20—60 | | |
Tissue	1	2	3—6	7—9	Group a dogs	Group b dogs	Group a dogs	Group b dogs	Group c dogs
Leukocytes	0/14	4/13	15/15	10/10	10/10	0/10	10/10	0/9	0/2
Conjunctival swab	0/6	0/6	1/8	9/9	8/10	2/10	7/8	0/10	0/2
Lymphatic system									
Spleen	0/5	2/5	8/8	8/8	6/6	1/6	12/12	0/12	0/2
Thymus	0/5	1/5	8/8	6/6	5/5	2/6	5/5	1/6	0/2
Bone marrow	0/5	1/5	8/8	6/6	4/4	1/5	3/3	0/4	—
Tonsils	1/5	1/5	7/8	6/6	5/5	0/5	6/6	0/5	—
Lymph nodes									
Bronchial	2/5	4/5	8/8	6/6	5/5	0/6	8/8	0/4	—
Retropharyngeal	0/5	2/5	7/8	6/6	4/4	0/6	6/6	0/4	—
Mesenteric	0/5	0/5	8/8	6/6	5/5	1/6	12/12	0/10	0/2
Alimentary tract									
Pharynx	0/3	0/3	3/3	5/5	5/5	1/6	6/6	0/4	—
Salivary gland	—	—	1/6	5/5	5/5	0/4	10/12	0/4	—
Esophagus	—	—	0/2	4/5	4/4	1/6	4/4	0/5	0/1
Stomach	—	—	0/2	5/5	4/4	2/6	4/4	1/6	1/2
Small intestine	0/5	0/5	7/8	5/5	5/5	1/6	12/12	1/10	0/2
Pancreas	—	—	1/6	4/5	4/5	0/4	9/12	1/7	0/1
Liver	0/2	1/3	2/4	4/4	4/4	0/4	8/8	—	—
Respiratory tract									
Trachea	—	—	—	3/3	2/2	0/3	—	0/3	—
Lungs	0/5	0/5	4/8	5/5	5/5	0/4	12/12	0/10	0/2
Urogenital tract									
Kidney	—	—	1/5	3/5	3/3	0/4	8/8	0/8	0/2
Bladder	—	—	0/5	4/5	4/4	1/6	5/5	1/8	1/2
Ovaries	—	—	0/2	0/2	0/1	—	0/3	0/1	—
Oviduct	—	—	0/2	2/2	1/1	—	3/3	0/1	—
Uterus	—	—	0/4	2/2	1/1	0/1	5/5	0/4	0/1
Vagina	—	—	0/2	2/2	1/1	—	3/3	0/2	—
Testes	—	—	0/1	1/1	1/2	—	4/6	0/4	—
Prostate gland	—	—	0/1	1/1	1/2	—	5/6	0/2	—
Endocrine system									
Pituitary gland	—	—	0/6	3/3	3/3	0/3	9/11	1/7	2/2
Pineal body	—	—	—	—	—	—	4/4	—	—
Thyroid gland	—	—	0/6	3/3	5/5	1/5	11/12	0/5	0/2
Parathyroid gland	—	—	0/4	1/1	4/4	0/3	6/7	0/3	0/1
Adrenal gland	—	—	1/4	3/3	1/1	—	7/10	0/4	0/1
Brain									
Meninges	—	—	0/5	1/5	4/5	0/6	12/12	0/11	0/2
Cerebellum	—	—	0/5	0/5	4/5	0/6	11/12	1/11	2/2
Cerebrum	—	—	—	0/5	1/3	0/2	9/12	0/11	2/2
Brain stem	—	—	—	0/5	1/3	0/2	10/12	0/11	2/2
Spinal cord	—	—	—	0/5	—	—	7/10	—	—
Skin									
Eyelid	—	0/2	3/3	5/5	5/5	1/6	6/6	0/6	0/2
Foot pad	—	—	0/3	5/5	4/4	1/6	4/5	2/10	2/2

Group *a* dogs with serum antibody titer 1 : 10 or less; group *b* dogs = dogs with serum antibody titer 1 : 100 or greater without clinical signs; and group *c* dogs = dogs with serum antibody titer 1 : 100 or greater with convulsions.

Numerator = number of dogs with virus in tissue; denominator = number of dogs examined.

Reprinted with permission from: APPEL, M. J. G.: Pathogenesis of Canine Distemper. Amer. J. vet. Res., **30**, 1167 (1969).

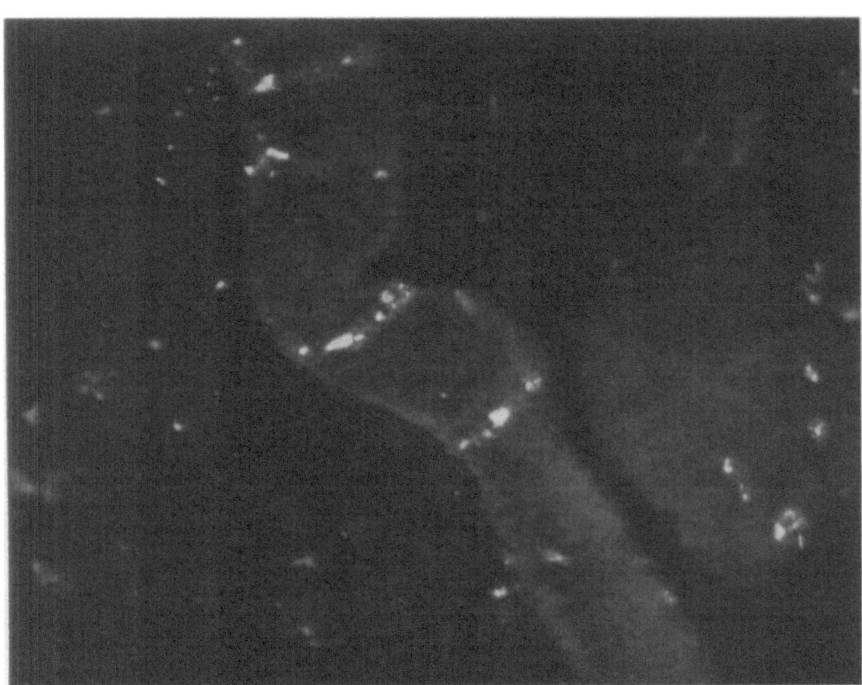

Fig. 14. Viral antigen in epithelium of gall bladder of dog 9 days after it was exposed to aerosol of canine distemper virus (× 250). Reprinted with permission from: APPEL, M. J. G.: Amer. J. vet. Res **30**, 1167 (1969)

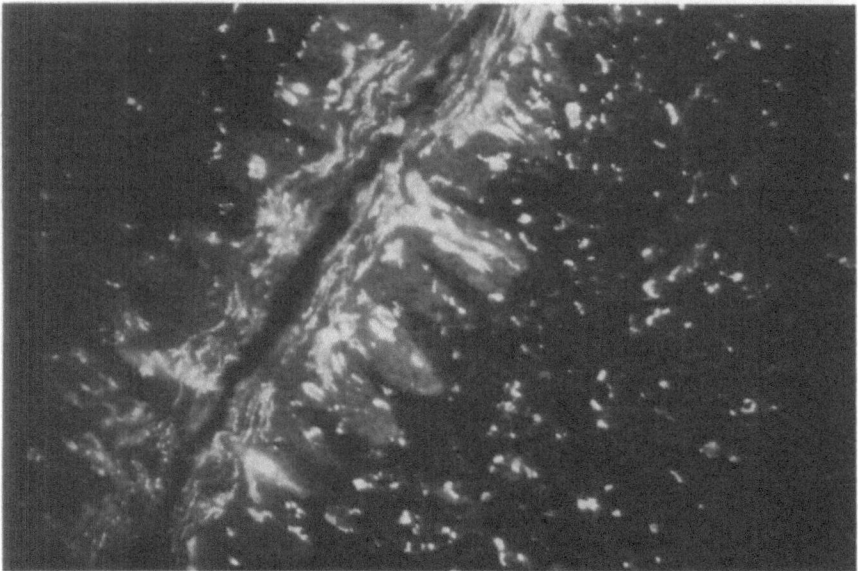

Fig. 15. Fluorescent epithelial and interstitial cells in esophagus of dog 21 days after it was exposed to aerosol of canine distemper virus (× 100). Reprinted with permission from: APPEL, M. J. G.: Amer. J. vet. Res. **30**, 1167 (1969)

ed in meningeal macrophages 9 days PI, then in cells in perivascular position, in ependymal cells, and later in glial cells and in neurons. These dogs died 3—4 weeks PI, some with convulsions. Serum and cerebrospinal fluid (CSF) had no or low levels of SN antibody.

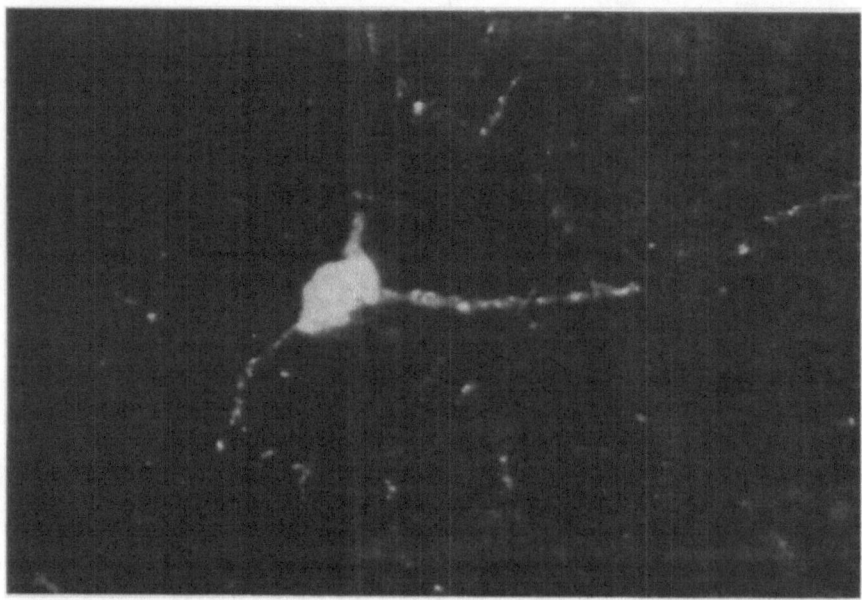

Fig. 16. Fluorescent granules in cytoplasm and axons, and dense fluorescent bodies in the nucleus of a neuron in cerebrum of a dog euthanatized 28 days after it was exposed to aerosol of canine distemper (× 250). Reprinted with permission from: APPEL, M. J. G.: Amer. J. vet. Res. **30**, 1167 (1969)

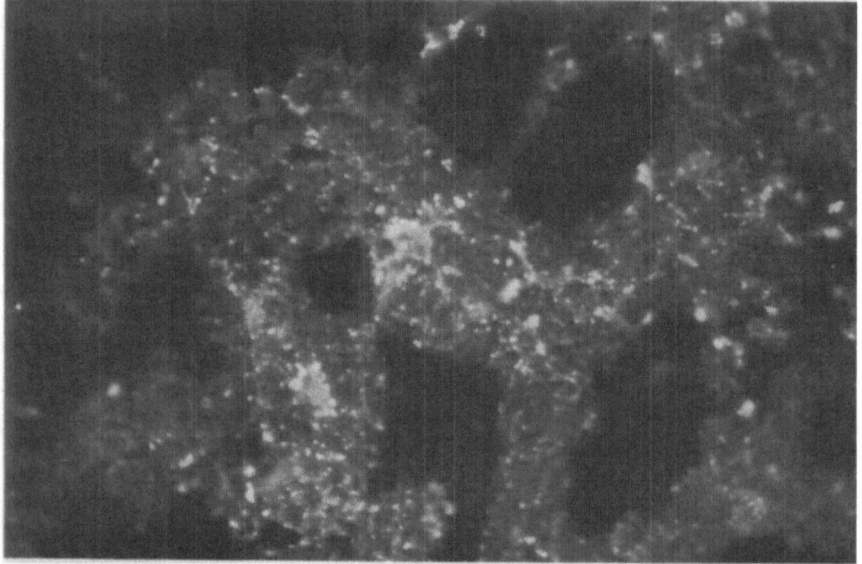

Fig. 17. Extensive fluorescence in cerebellar white matter of dog which had demyelinating encephalitis 31 days after it was exposed to aerosol of canine distemper virus (× 250). Reprinted with permission from: APPEL, M. J. G.: Amer. J. vet. Res. **30**, 1167 (1969)

The exception were 2 dogs which did form antibody and appeared healthy until they had convulsions and died with demyelinating encephalitis 41 and 60 days PI. Distribution of viral antigen in these dogs and presence of SN antibody in serum and CSF was similar to cases of "late" distemper encephalitis in random dogs (APPEL, 1970). Serum and CSF had high titer SN antibody. Viral antigen was restricted to neurons (Fig. 16) and white matter (Fig. 17) of the brain, to pituitary gland, a few epithelial cells in alimentary, respiratory, and urogenital tract, and to footpad gland and epidermal cells (Fig. 18).

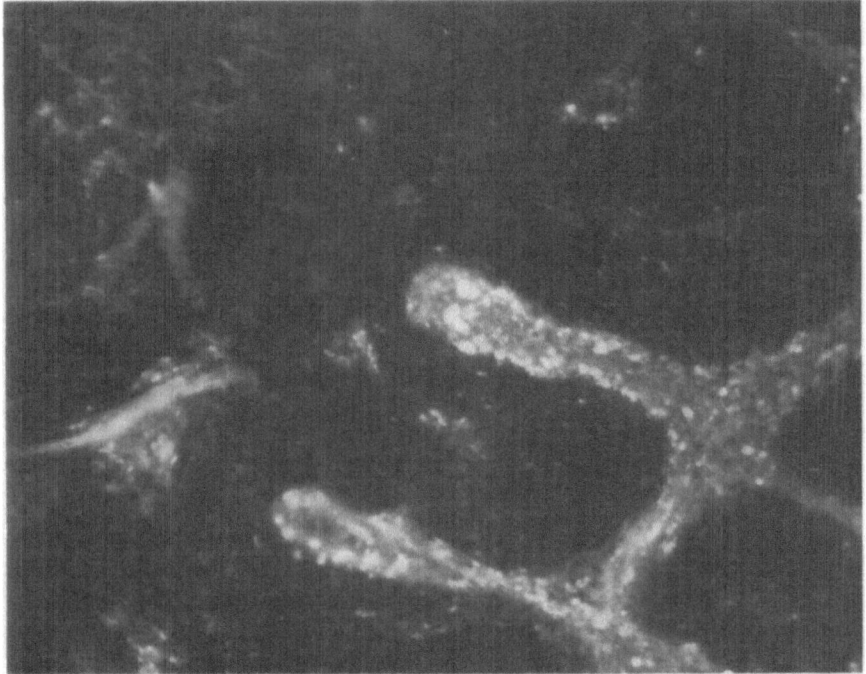

Fig. 18. Viral antigen in foot pad epidermis of a moribund dog with canine distemper (× 100). Reprinted with permission from: APPEL, M. J. G.: Amer. J. vet. Res. **30**, 1167 (1969)

Other experimental data (PECKHAM, 1967) likewise indicated that CDV reached the brain through meninges and cerebrospinal fluid producing virus encephalitis. The development of demyelination in CD encephalitis will be discussed in the Pathology section (cf. p. 62).

4. Excretion of Distemper Virus

Dogs with an acute systemic infection and generalized virus distribution shed virus in practically every excretion. CARRÉ (1905) and later GREEN (1926) demonstrated the presence of distemper virus in filtered nasal exudate. GORHAM and BRANDLY (1953) exposed ferrets and mink to distemper virus by aerosol. Nasal exudate and saliva contained infectious virus 5 days after exposure and virus persisted until death in ferrets and up to 51 days in mink. Swabs of conjunctival exudate collected on the 21st and 30th day revealed virus. GORHAM (1968) found virus in nasal washings from dogs up to 28 days after virus exposure. BINDRICH (1951 a) found distemper virus in the urine several days after viremia occurred. This observation was confirmed by GORHAM (1968). Distemper virus isolation from feces was not always achieved (GORHAM, 1960), but virus spread did occur from feces of dogs with acute distemper.

B. Immunity

1. Active Immunity

Dogs surviving virulent CDV infection are generally considered to have a lifelong immunity. This is difficult to evaluate since exposure to street virus probably occurs frequently in city dogs. Duration of immunity for at least 7 years was found by GILLESPIE (unpublished), who kept CD immune dogs in isolation for this period of time and then challenged with virulent CDV. However, it is known that occasionally older dogs in urban populations with a history of previous vaccination many years ago develop CD and die. Immunity challenge in dogs has been difficult to evaluate since contact exposure to virulent CDV or parenteral inoculation does not result in a 100 per cent morbidity or mortality. A reliable method for challenging CD immunity in dogs was produced by inoculating intracerebrally brain-adapted strains of CDV (BINDRICH, 1954; GILLESPIE and RICKARD, 1956). Ferrets respond with an almost 100 per cent mortality to virulent CDV and they often have been used for immunity tests. CABASSO et al. (1957) reported persistence of immunity in ferrets after vaccination with egg-adapted virus for at least 5.5 years and GORHAM (1960) showed protection for at least 4 years.

More studies on duration of immunity have been based on presence of neutralizing antibody. Concurrent with CD immunity in dogs appears the production of neutralizing antibody which serves presently as the only *in vitro* index for immunity in dogs. A titer of 1 : 100 or greater can be correlated with absolute protection against intracerebral or aerosol challenge with the Snyder Hill strain of CDV (GILLESPIE et al., 1958). This should not be confused with the production of high antibody titers in some dogs during infection which later develop nervous manifestations of CD (APPEL, 1969). Dogs with a titer of 1 : 20 or less were found to be fully susceptible to CDV (GILLESPIE et al., 1958). However, there are exceptions. Dogs with little or no neutralizing antibody titer may be clinically protected as shown by GILLESPIE (1965). Dogs after vaccination with inactivated CD virus or with measles virus have little or no measurable circulating CD antibody. When they are challenged with virulent CDV they are protected and react with an anamnestic antibody response. The amount of neutralizing antibody, therefore, is only a relative index for immunity to CDV.

2. Neutralizing Antibody

Neutralization tests with CDV antiserum have been studied extensively. For many years the inhibition of egg-adapted CDV growth in embryonated hen eggs has been most reliable and has been used in many laboratories. After CABASSO et al. (1951) first reported a qualitative test for neutralizing antibodies, a quantitative test has been developed (ANDERSSON, 1954; BAKER et al., 1954; IMAGAWA et al., 1954; MANTOVANI, 1954 b; SCHINDLER, 1954; KARZON, 1955; GORHAM,

1957 a; Gillespie *et al.*, 1958). The specificity of this neutralization test was demonstrated by Gillespie *et al.* (1958) and Karzon *et al.* (1961) and the relationship between virus and antibody levels was observed as a linear slope (Fig. 19). A ten-fold virus variation resulted in eight-fold serum titer variation according to Baker *et al.* (1954). These results have been questioned by Schroeder and Bordt (1962).

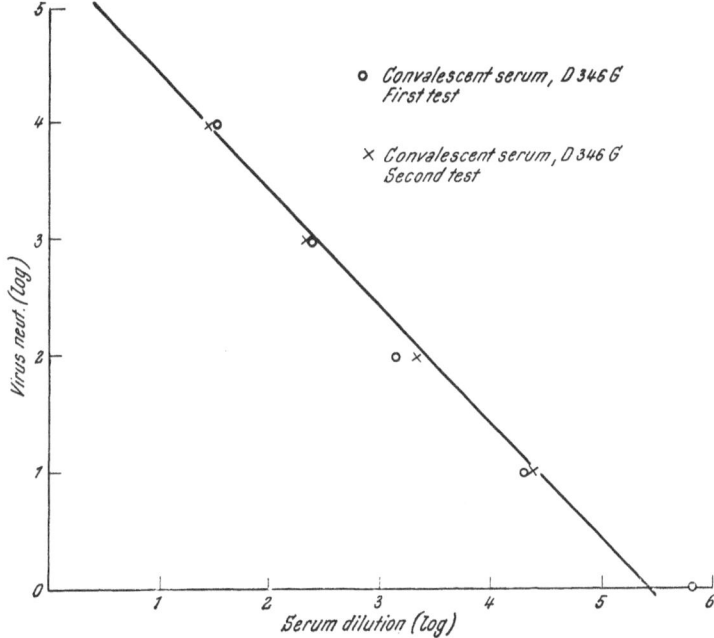

Fig. 19. Slope of neutralization titers (calculated by method of Reed and Muench) against egg-adapted canine distemper virus when checked by the chick embryo neutralization test. Reprinted with permission from: Gillespie et al.: Cornell Vet. 48, 103 (1958)

A wide variety of different incubation times and temperatures, dilution steps and virus doses have been employed in the egg CDV neutralization test. Their errors were discussed by Lo *et al.* (1965). Optimal temperature and time for a test in which thermal virus inactivation was minimal, and the virus-antibody association, reached an equilibrium in an adequately short period of time, was found to be 16 hours at 25° C (Lo *et al.*, 1965 a). For quantitative studies, the conventional test with serial serum dilutions was found to be superior to a single dilution test which was more sensitive for the detection of minimal quantities of antibody (Lo *et al.*, 1965 b).

At a symposium on CD (J.A.V.M.A., June 1966) a Committee on Standardized Reagents and Test Procedures made recommendations for the standardization of this test. The recommendations were based principally on the statistical evaluation tests by Robson *et al.* (1961).

Various tissue culture systems may be used for CD neutralization tests. The tissue culture-adapted CDV strain of Rockborn (1958 a) has been used in dog kidney cell cultures in several laboratories; however, this test did not appear to be as sensitive as the egg test. A plaque reduction test has been described by Karzon and BUSSEL (1959) using egg-adapted CDV in chick embryo fibroblast cultures with an agar overlay. GOURLAY (1970) used egg-adapted virus in Vero cells with a carboxymethyl cellulose overlay for plaque reduction tests. Vero cells appear promising for CDV neutralization test (BROWN, unpublished). Serum neutralization tests can be made in microplates with egg-adapted CDV in Vero cells (APPEL, unpublished).

Neutralization tests can be performed in mice and suckling hamsters by use of adapted CDV strains for these species. CARLSTRÖM (1958, 1962) considered the mouse system to be very sensitive. Before the egg or tissue culture systems became available, dogs and ferrets were used (LAIDLAW and DUNKIN, 1931).

Serum neutralizing antibodies in dogs appeared first 8 or 9 days after aerosol exposure to virulent CDV (APPEL, 1969) in the conventional *in ovo* test. Maximal antibody levels were found 2 to 4 weeks after exposure which were usually between 1 : 300 and 1 : 3000. There seem to be differences in response to different strains (ROCKBORN, 1958 b; BINN, personal communication). After parenteral inoculation of virulent or adapted virus, serum antibody usually can be detected 2 days earlier. (ROCKBORN, 1957 a; GILLESPIE et al., 1958; BAKER et al., 1959; JOHNSTON et al., 1959; PIERCY et al., 1960; YORK et al., 1960; THOMAS et al., 1963). Peak levels of serum antibody after injection of vaccine virus are usually between 1 : 100 and 1 : 1000, slightly below levels after virulent virus exposure. In ferrets, LO et al. (1965 b) found CD neutralizing antibody only 8 days post-immunization in the conventional *in ovo* test, while in the single dilution test, virus neutralization was observed on the 4th day.

Duration of neutralizing antibody in kennel dogs after vaccination with the Lederle strain has been studied by ROBSON et al. (1959). Approximately 96 per cent of dogs had antibody titers above 1 : 100 four weeks after vaccination. One year later, approximately 33 per cent of the dogs had neutralizing antibody titers below 1 : 100, and 2 years later another 33 per cent had reduced antibody titers below 1 : 100. KEEBLE (1932) reported logarithmic antibody declination at the rate of 0.5 $\log_{10}$ every 6 or 7 months. PIERCY (1961) recorded neutralizing antibody in 6 of 8 dogs maintained in isolation for 3 to 4 years. Neutralizing antibody was present in 89 per cent of 64 dogs 2 to 6 years after vaccination with egg-adapted virus (PRYDIE, 1966).

According to test results from the Diagnostic Laboratory, Cornell University (BOYER, 1966; personal communication) approximately 10 per cent of 700 adult female dogs in the Eastern United States had no demonstrable neutralizing antibody and an additional 10 per cent had titers less than 1 : 100. All of these dogs had been vaccinated previously against CD, and serum samples were sent for a CD nomograph determination.

With minor differences, there seems to be a general agreement on serological results in these studies. Some difference appeared since some authors reported on levels of antibody and others on presence of antibody. For a practical purpose, interpretation of these results raise the question to which we have no definite answer: "Is revaccination necessary for protection in dogs and if so, when and how often." As mentioned previously, little is known about the immune status in dogs lacking CD neutralizing antibody. Some answers are given with the study of heterotypic vaccination with measles virus, which will be discussed in that section (cf. p. 71). For greater safety, annual vaccination of all dogs has been recommended in a symposium on canine distemper immunization (GILLESPIE et al., 1966).

Electrophoretic patterns of CD neutralizing antibody were reported from serum and cerebrospinal fluid (CSF). The main fraction in serum appeared in the gamma globulin fraction; however, differentiations between Ig G and Ig M have not been made (POLSON and MALHERBE, 1952; GENTILE et al., 1960; MEBUS and COLES, 1965). These authors and SNOW et al. (1966) also found an increase in the alpha-2 fraction during initial and advanced stages of CD and a decrease in albumin. MEBUS and COLES (1965) considered the increase in the alpha-2 and the decrease in the albumin fraction to be nonspecific, since both occurred in stress reactions and tissue injury under a number of different conditions.

CD neutralizing antibody can be found in the CSF of dogs with demyelinating CD encephalitis (APPEL, 1969; CUTLER and AVERILL, 1969). Of 16 such dogs studied (CUTLER and AVERILL, 1969) 10 had a marked elevation of CSF Ig G concentration, 4 had a moderate elevation and 2 had a low concentration. 6 of the 10 dogs with a marked elevation had also an increase in the CSF Ig M fraction. In a control group, 10 of 11 dogs had a low concentration of CSF Ig G and the other had a moderate elevation.

3. Complement-Fixing Antibody

The complement fixation test has been used much longer than the serum neutralization test for the study of CD antibodies (LAIDLAW and DUNKIN, 1931). Complement-fixing antibodies developed 3 to 4 weeks after initial infection but the CF antibody only persisted for a few weeks thereafter (MANSI, 1955; KARZON et al., 1961; MORRIS et al., 1955). Because CF antibody disappeared relatively soon after an initial infection, this test offered a means by which a recent infection could be diagnosed. A second injection of virus elicited the production of CF antibody quickly with the peak titer attained at approximately 7 days after inoculation (LAIDLAW and DUNKIN, 1931; DRÄGER and SCHINDLER, 1951 a; MANSI, 1955; KARZON et al., 1961). Dogs given three injections of formalin-inactivated dog spleen virus at bi-weekly intervals had detectable CF titers 29 days later; however, the titers decreased rapidly and were not detectable at 2.5 months (KARZON et al., 1961). When these dogs were challenged with virulent Snyder Hill CDV 3.5 months after the first injection of inactivated virus vaccine, they developed unusually high CF titers in 4 to 8 days that persisted at a significant level for the remaining 7 months that they were kept in semi-isolation.

4. Antibody Inhibiting Measles Hemagglutinins

WATERSON et al. (1963) noticed an inhibition by CD antiserum of monkey erythrocyte agglutination with measles virus hemagglutinin. Hemagglutination was not inhibited when complete measles virus was used, but it was inhibited by CD antiserum when measles virus was treated with Tween 80 and ether, which separated the viral envelopes into small, more uniform hemagglutinin. However, not all CD antisera inhibited hemagglutination. HI antibodies were detectable in dogs immunized with attenuated Rockborn CDV, but not in dogs after exposure to the virulent Snyder Hill strain (WATERSON et al., 1963; ENDERS-RUCKLE, 1964; NORBY, 1967). Serum neutralizing antibody titers were similar in both groups.

5. Passive Immunity by Maternal Antibody

Neutralizing antibody to CDV is transferred from the dam to the progeny *in utero* and by colostral feeding (GILLESPIE *et al.*, 1958). Approximately 2.9 per cent is transferred *in utero* and the combined placental-colostral antibody amount is equivalent to an average of 77 per cent of the bitches serum (GILLESPIE *et al.*, 1958) (Fig. 20). Limited studies suggested that the major transfer of colostral antibody occurred within the first day of life. The half life of the maternally transferred antibody was 8.4 days (GILLESPIE *et al.*, 1958).

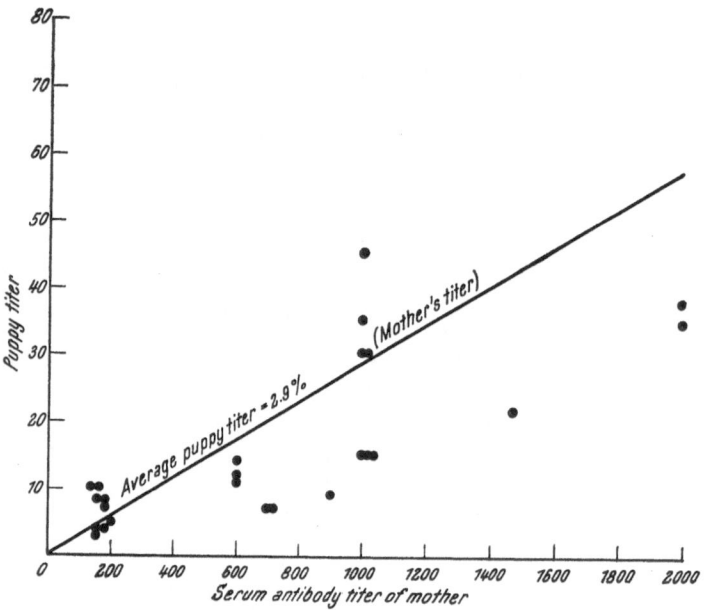

Fig. 20. Relationship between titer of mother and antibodies acquired by progeny through placental transfer. Reprinted with permission from: GILLESPIE *et al.*: Cornell Vet. 48, 103 (1958)

Serum-neutralization tests in embryonated hen eggs with 300 EID_{50} of Onderstepoort virus indicated that puppies with maternal antibody titers less than 1 : 20 were clearly susceptible to challenge with virulent Snyder Hill strain of CDV and those with antibody titers above 1 : 100 were definitely immune to challenge (GILLESPIE *et al.*, 1958). There was an increasing susceptibility with decreasing maternal antibody titers. Fifty per cent of puppies with titers between 1 : 30 and 1 : 40 were susceptible. Puppies from immune mothers could not be actively immunized until they had lost their colostral protection. This applied to *in utero* transferred antibody as well as to the combined placental-colostral antibody. Thus, puppies from a mother with a high antibody titer which had not received colostrum were protected against challenge for 1 week after birth, but not for 2 weeks. Until these studies were conducted, infant puppies were considered immunologically incompetent and, therefore, incapable of producing good CD antibody titers when vaccinated early in life. It is now known that failures to immunize puppies with potent virus were due to maternal antibody protection (Fig. 21). An effect of age on distemper antibody production was not discernible in these studies. The results obtained by CARMICHAEL *et al.* (1962) with maternal immunity to infectious canine hepatitis virus were remarkably similar to those obtained with CD. Furthermore, susceptible puppies responded well serologically to infectious canine hepatitis vaccine virus at one day of age which indicates that the infant puppy is competent immunologically at an early age.

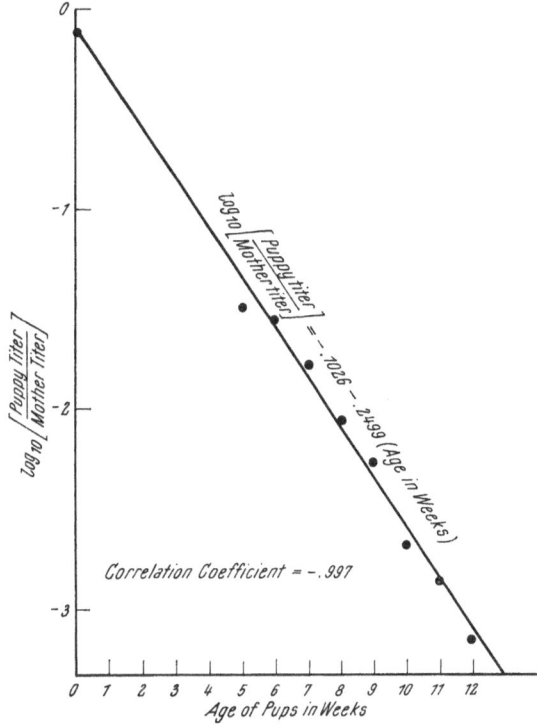

Fig. 21. Relationship between age of puppy and the puppy's titer as a percentage of the mother's titer. Reprinted with permission from: GILLESPIE *et al.*: Cornell Vet. 48, 103 (1958)

From experimental data in which the neutralization test in embryonated chicken eggs and the Snyder Hill virulent strain for immunity challenge were used to evaluate maternal protection to CD in puppies, a nomograph was devised to predict the earliest age at which to vaccinate puppies, based upon the serum antibody titer of the bitch (GILLESPIE *et al.*, 1958). Only 82 per cent of the puppies from immune mothers developed titers greater than 1 : 100 when egg-adapted vaccine virus was used in the first field trials based on the nomograph in contrast to the anticipated 98 per cent that was attained when virulent test virus was used in susceptible puppies. The nomograph was then revised (Fig. 22) by adding an additional week to the predicted time when virulent virus was employed; and 96 per cent of the puppies tested unter field conditions developed active immunity after inoculation with egg-adapted vaccine virus (BAKER *et al.*, 1959).

The nomograph procedure has been in use in the United States for at least 10 years. The service is used primarily to assist veterinarians in their distemper vaccination programs where the progeny of valuable breeding dogs is involved.

6. Immunological Relationship between Canine Distemper and Other Viruses

a) Canine Distemper and Measles Virus

Measles virus induces both MV and CDV antibody in various species, although the CDV antibody appears in low levels. Dogs inoculated with MV are protected against later challenge with virulent CDV even if measurable CDV antibody is not present. Canine distemper virus usually induces only CDV antibody in various species, but exceptions were found. Convincing protection from clinical measles

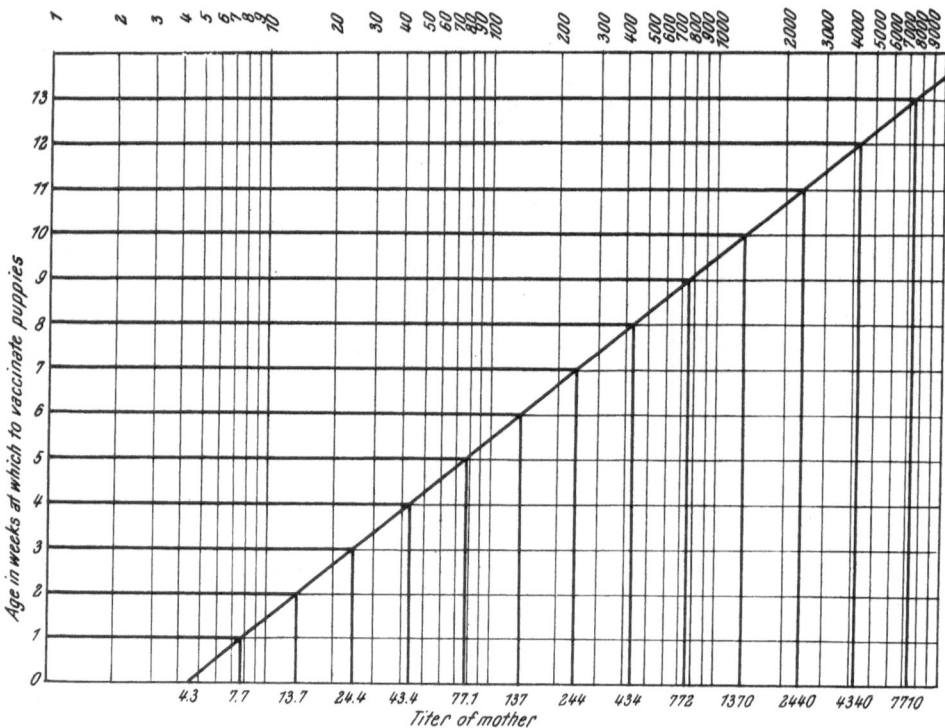

Fig. 22. The distemper nomograph that predicts the earliest age at which to vaccinate pups — based on antibody titer of the bred female. Reprinted with permission from: BAKER et al.: Cornell Vet. **49**, 158 (1959)

in human volunteers was not produced by CDV. The immunological and serological (Table 5) relationship between CDV and MV has been summarized recently by IMAGAWA (1968).

The first suggestion of a possible relationship between CDV and MV arose from histopathological studies of infant pneumonitis by PINKERTON et al. (1945) who noticed similarities in the pathologic response to these viruses in their natural hosts. BRYAN (1928), NICOLLE (1931), and ADAMS (1941) previously had thought that CDV may produce pneumonitis in man. This led ADAMS (1953), KARZON (1955), CARLSTRÖM (1956) and PRIER et al. (1956) to search for serological evidence of CD antibodies in humans. They found CD neutralizing antibodies widespread in the USA population. Antibody was transmitted across the placental barrier and was lost when a child reached 6 to 20 months of age. By the age of 10 years, practically all children had CD neutralizing antibodies in significant titers. Consequently, the authors concluded that their data were typical for a widespread infectious agent. HOPPER (1959 b) reported on CD neutralizing antibody in human serum from different countries.

CARLSTRÖM (1957) and ADAMS and IMAGAWA (1957) independently reported a probable relationship between CDV and MV by the use of serological tests. Mouse-adapted CDV was neutralized by human convalescent measles sera and measles antiserum prepared in ferrets, but not by sera from the acute phase or pre-infection [ADAMS and IMAGAWA (1957) and IMAGAWA et al. (1960)]. KARZON (1962)

Table 5. *Heterologous Antibody in Measles, Rinderpest, and Canine Distemper Antiserums*

Antiserums	Serologic test[1]	Antibody response					
		Before inoculation, or in acute stage			In serums from convalescent animals		
		Measles	Rinder-pest	Canine distemper	Measles	Rinder-pest	Canine distemper
Measles (43 to 22 ID monkey)	CF	<2	<10	<4	512	40	<4
	Neut.	<4	<1	<5	17,80	2	8
Rinderpest (rabbit 9)	CF	<2	<10	<4	<2	320	<4
	Neut.	<4	<1	<5	16	4	<5
Rinderpest (steer 2159)	CF	<2	<10	<4	<2	40	<4
	Neut.	<4	<1	<5	12	3	<5
Canine distemper (B 60—66 dog)	CF	<2	<10	<4	16	320	16
	Neut.	<4	<1	<5	4	1	1,280

[1] CF = Complement-fixation test
Neut. = Virus-neutralization test
ID = Infective doses

Reprinted with permission from: DELAY et al.: Amer. J. vet. Res., **26**, 1359 (1965).

plotted the development of measles and distemper antibody responses in naturally occurring measles cases in children. Both antibodies were acquired with the measles antibody appearing between the 5th and 7th day after the onset of illness. In contrast, the distemper-neutralizing antibody appeared later and the titers were lower. The titers of both antibodies persisted for six months with no loss. Monkeys infected with measles virus reacted similarly. It is now generally believed that measles infection is solely responsible for the presence of distemper-neutralizing antibody in humans. There is no clear evidence that distemper virus replicates in man (BLACK and ROSEN, 1962). A febrile response in young cynomolgous monkeys after virulent CDV inoculation was observed by DELAY et al. (1965).

The relationships of MV and CDV in other animal species were more complex. Monkeys infected with measles virus reacted like humans and regularly produced neutralizing antibodies to distemper and measles. Infection of ferrets, rabbits, and guinea pigs with MV produced measles-neutralizing antibody but only low distemper-neutralizing antibody titers in some of the animals (IMAGAWA et al.,

1960; KARZON, 1960). Dogs after one inoculation of MV produced homologous CF and neutralizing antibody only (DELAY et al., 1965). After 2 inoculation, slow levels of CD neutralizing antibody were also found (ROBERTS, 1965). An anamnestic MV neutralizing antibody response was induced in dogs with CDV after MV inoculation (ROBERTS, 1965; BITTLE, 1970). Protection studies with MV against CD challenge were made in dogs by WARREN et al. (1960), MOURA, and WARREN (1961), GILLESPIE and KARZON (1961). In experiments by the latter investigators, some dogs immunized with MV were injected intracerebrally with the neurogenic Snyder Hill strain and all withstood the challenge. These challenge experiments clearly demonstrated protection despite little or no distemper-neutralizing antibody. There was correlation between protection and anamnestic CDV antibody response after challenge with CDV (see also: Heterotypic Virus Vaccines, p. 71). Ferrets inoculated with MV were partially protected against later challenge with virulent CDV (ADAMS and IMAGAWA, 1957).

When CDV was inoculated into various species, production of MV antibody has been found less frequently and protection against MV was less effective. Dogs hyperimmunized against CDV had no MV neutralizing antibody (KARZON, 1962; DELAY et al., 1965; ROBERTS, 1965). However, MV stimulated an anamnestic CDV antibody response in CD immune dogs (ROBERTS, 1965). Rabbits and chickens after CDV inoculation produced CDV antibody in all animals but very little MV antibody in a few animals (KARZON, 1965). Monkeys (SCHWARZ et al., 1960; DELAY et al., 1965) and cattle (DELAY et al., 1965) reacted in a similar way. Human volunteers have been inoculated with CDV and they produced low titer of CDV antibody only (MILLIAN et al., 1960; SCHWARZ et al., 1960) or CDV and MV antibody (HOEKENGA et al., 1960).

There has been some evidence of clinical protection against natural measles infection in human beings after immunization with CDV but the results did not warrant its use as a vaccine for man (ADAMS et al., 1959; HOEKENGA et al., 1960).

The biological test system used to detect the presence of neutralizing antibody appeared to be important. For example, the mouse-neutralization test was more sensitive for measuring heterologous reactions than the tissue culture or chick embryo neutralization test (CARLSTRÖM, 1958, 1959, 1962). CDV antiserum prepared in rabbits neutralized mouse adapted measles virus (CARLSTRÖM, 1958). Tissue culture-adapted measles virus was neutralized by CDV hyperimmune serum prepared in ferrets but only in low dilution (IMAGAWA et al., 1960).

Best evidence for a group specific complement-fixing antigen has been brought by WATERSON et al. (1963) who disrupted measles virions with Tween-ether. The purified non-hemagglutinating nucleoprotein fixed complement with CDV and MV antibody. Complete virions gave very little heterologous response. BECH (1960), WARREN et al. (1960), and CARLSTRÖM (1962) found cross-complement fixing reactions with serum after natural human measles infection and experimental CD infection.

Hemagglutination-inhibition (HI) was found with some CDV antisera when measles virus was treated with Tween-ether which disrupted the viral envelopes into more uniform hemagglutinin (WATERSON et al., 1963; ENDERS-RUCKLE, 1964). These HI antibodies were only found in dogs immunized with Rockborn's attenuated CDV but not in dogs recovered from the virulent Snyder Hill strain.

b) Canine Distemper and Rinderpest Virus

Rinderpest virus (RV) may or may not induce CDV antibody in various species, but dogs inoculated with RV are protected against later challenge with virulent CDV. Canine distemper virus usually induces RV antibody of low titer in various species, but cattle may or may not be protected with CDV against later challenge with virulent RV. Results on immunological and serological (Table 5) relationships between CDV and RV have been summarized recently by IMAGAWA (1968) and PLOWRIGHT (1968).

An immunological relationship between CDV and RV was found by POLDING and SIMPSON (1957) and GORET (1957) within the same year when a CDV-MV relationship was described. Experimental work was based on the observation that dogs fed on RV infected meat were resistant to exposure of CDV. Rinderpest virus apparently replicates well in dogs producing viremia with subsequent homologous antibody formation. This has been found with virulent strains of RV (POLDING and SIMPSON, 1957; SCOTT and BROWN, 1958; POLDING et al., 1959; DELAY et al., 1965) and with lapinized strains of RV (MORNET et al., 1960). When these infected dogs were challenged later with virulent CDV, they did not develop clinical disease in spite of the absence of CD antibody at the time of challenge. It must be assumed that protection was induced by an anamnestic CD antibody response similar to the anamnestic response after MV inoculation. However, RV appeared to replicate more readily in dogs than MV; therefore, smaller doses of RV than MV were probably sufficient for protection. Protection was not likely induced by viral interference since ferrets were protected one year after RV inoculation (GORET et al., 1960).

Ferrets did not always produce homologous antibody after RV inoculation and they were not always protected against CDV challenge (GORET et al., 1958; MORNET et al., 1959, 1960). Perhaps protection in ferrets was more dose-dependent than in dogs. Time between inoculations appeared to be important. Ferrets challenged with CDV 9 or more days after RV were always protected (GORET et al., 1960).

Passive immunization of dogs (POLDING et al., 1959) or ferrets (GORET et al., 1960) with hyperimmune RV antiserum was unsuccessful, although in vitro neutralization was found by some authors (GORET et al., 1959; MORNET et al., 1960; IMAGAWA et al., 1960) but not by others (MORNET et al., 1960; DELAY et al., 1965) using different test systems. In agar gel diffusion tests, spur formation was seen when hyperimmune RV antiserum prepared in rabbits was diffused against CDV and RV antigens, indicating a difference in antigens (WHITE et al., 1961).

Monkeys, like dogs, did not produce CDV antibody after RV inoculation (DELAY et al., 1965). Distemper virus apparently does not replicate as well in cattle as RV does in dogs. CDV induced protection against RV in cattle appeared more dose-dependent and was only induced with large doses of CDV (MORNET et al., 1959) similar to MV in dogs. Also, 12—18 days were required between CDV and RV inoculations for reliable protection (MORNET et al., 1960). Again, an anamnestic RV antibody response probably caused protection which was still found 6 months after CDV infection (GILBERT et al., 1960). Protection was induced with virulent or avianized virus (GORET et al., 1958; MORNET et al., 1960). However, protection was not found by all authors. POLDING et al. (1959) gave repeated doses of CDV to cattle which did not resist RV challenge later. Production of CDV antibody in cattle after inoculation was used as an indicator for protection against RV (GILBERT et al., 1960). This observation was not confirmed in another study. DELAY et al. (1965) reported presence of neutralizing antibody in 5 of 6 and CF antibody in one of 6 cattle 24 days after inoculation with virulent CDV. All cattle died when challenged at that time with the Kabete 0 strain of Virulent RV.

Rabbits were not protected by virulent or avianized CDV against lapinized RV, even when large doses, repeated inoculations and adjuvants were employed (GORET et al., 1960; MORNET et al., 1960; PLOWRIGHT, 1962).

Young cynomolgous monkeys after inoculation with virulent CDV developed CDV neutralizing and RV complement-fixing antibody (DELAY, 1965).

In vitro neutralization of RV by CDV antiserum was found to a limited degree (POLDING and SIMPSON, 1957; GORET et al., 1960; MORNET et al., 1960; VILLEMONT et al., 1961; DELAY et al., 1965). In agar gel diffusion tests, fusing lines were seen when hyperimmune CDV antiserum prepared in dogs diffused against RV and CDV antigens indicating identity (WHITE et al., 1961).

C. Variation

As GORHAM (1960) stated, "Knowledge of any antigenic differences between isolates of a virus is important in epizootiological studies and in the choice of vaccine strains". There is a general agreement today that immunological strain variations in CDV do not exist in MV and RV. Various strains of CDV were studied earlier by LAIDLAW and DUNKIN (1928 a) with these points in mind. Their observations showed that recovered ferrets or dogs were immune against subsequent challenges with other strains. They thought minor differences may exist between strains because some ferrets given inactivated CDV vaccine were later susceptible to virulent virus which was probably due to dose and time differentials.

MACINTYRE et al. (1948) presented a paper in England which created much interest and controversy. They stated that the typical nervous manifestations in dogs usually associated with CD was, in reality, caused by another agent. The new condition was termed "hard pad disease" of dogs because the outstanding pathologic alteration was hyperkeratosis of the foot pads and nose associated with demyelinating encephalitis. Their main thesis for a separate etiology was the prolonged incubation period of 17 days or longer in the ferret with tissues from "hard pad" cases as compared with the usual 10-day incubation period with regular strains of CDV. Their conclusions received considerable support by clinicians and some pathologists in the United States and England because it seemed like a valid reason for immunization failures with CD biologics. It has been discussed in many publications (COHRS, 1951; FANKHAUSER, 1951; SCHEITLIN et al., 1951; FENNER and SCHINDLER, 1952; MANSI, 1952; LARIN, 1954; GORHAM, 1960). The MACINTYRE postulation did not hold true. Immunological and serological identity of CDV and the "hard pad" agent was soon demonstrated (KOPROWSKI et al., 1950; DRÄGER and SCHINDLER, 1951; CABASSO and COX, 1952; CABASSO, 1952; GILLESPIE et al., 1958; POTEL and BINDRICH, 1958).

The prolonged incubation period in ferrets found by MACINTYRE et al. (1948) probably reflected low virus titers and presence of neutralizing antibody in tissues of dogs with "hard pad" disease, a chronic form of distemper. Prolonged incubation periods in CDV inoculated ferrets have been observed repeatedly (GREEN and CARLSON, 1945; MANSI, 1952; GORHAM, 1960; RECULARD and GUILLON, 1967). After serial passages in ferrets, the incubation period was reduced to the usual 8 to 14 days in all cases.

Cross-protection tests in dogs were performed by GILLESPIE and RICKARD (1956) with strains of CDV from various sources and origins. Dogs that received the Fromm Distemperiod, Buffalo "hard pad", egg-adapted Lederle, or egg-adapted Onderstepoort strains were immune to challenge with the Snyder Hill strain.

Table 6. *The Results of Some Cross Protection Tests Using Different Isolates of Distemper Virus*

Immunogenic isolate	References	Laidlaw-Dunkin Isolate	Green	Glasgow S 123	Wellcome Hard Pad	Delavan Mink	Lederle A	Lederle B	Available isolates of distemper encephalitis	Fromm	Snyder Hill	Buffalo	Haig Encephalitis	Rockborn Thun
Swedish	ROCKBORN, 1957 a	I[1]												
Raccoon 9[3]	CROOK and McNUTT, 1958	I												
Buffalo[2]	GILLESPIE and RICKARD, 1956										I			
Fromm	GILLESPIE and RICKARD, 1956										I			
Snyder Hill	GILLESPIE and RICKARD, 1956								I		I	I		
Lederle B[2, 3]	CABASSO and COX, 1952 GORHAM, 1954 GILLESPIE and RICKARD, 1956 ROCKBORN, 1958 b	I					I	I			I			I
Lederle A[3]	GORHAM, 1954	I							I					
Wisconsin FXNO[3]	GORHAM, 1954	I				I								
Wellcome Hard Pad	MANSI, 1952	I	I	I										
Green	MANSI, 1952	I		I	I									
Laidlaw-Dunkin	MANSI, 1952		I	I	I									
Onderstepoort[3, 4]	GILLESPIE and RICKARD, 1956 HAIG, 1956 BAKER et al., 1952	I									I		I	
Glasgow S 123	MANSI, 1952	I	I		I									

[1] Immune to challenge.
[2] Isolate from a dog exhibiting neurotropic signs.
[3] Egg-propagated distemper virus.
[4] The Onderstepoort virus is a variant derived from Green's Distemperoid.

Reprinted with permission from: GORHAM, JOHN R.: Canine Distemper. Advanc. vet. Sci., **6**, 287—351 (1960).

Furthermore, convalescent sera collected from dogs injected with any of the five strains neutralized the Onderstepoort and Lederle viruses in the hens' egg neutralization test for distemper.

The evidence presented by many investigators clearly showed that there was only one immunogenic type of CDV (GORHAM, 1960) (Table 6).

The variation of CDV pathogenicity from species to species ranges from a 100 per cent mortality in ferrets over an approximately 50 per cent mortality in dogs to an inapparent infection in cats (APPEL et al., 1971).

D. Clinicopathological Features

1. Clinical

Canine distemper has a worldwide distribution and is the most serious disease of dogs. It produces a wide variety of clinical symptoms in dogs that range from virtually no visible disease (GIBSON et al., 1965) to severe disease with high mortality. This inconsistency exists between and within litters of pups which have been exposed to the same strain of virus (LAIDLAW and DUNKIN, 1926 a; CORNWELL et al., 1965 a; APPEL, 1969). One explanation for this divergence is the early progressive antibody formation in some dogs, which leads to protection (APPEL, 1969 — see Pathogenesis). CDV causes destruction of lymphatic tissue early in the disease, affecting cells that are responsible for antibody formation, and producing a competitive process. Destruction of lymphatic tissue also appears to reduce host resistance to secondary agents, and secondary infections play an important role in the natural disease. Bacteria, Mycoplasma, protozoa, and other viruses can often be found to be complicating factors. Nutrition appears to influence the course of the disease (NEWBERNE, 1966; BRESNAHAN and NEWBERNE, 1968).

There have been many descriptions of clinical distemper in dogs. Only a few references shall be given here (CARRÉ, 1905; LAIDLAW and DUNKIN, 1926 a; MACINTYRE, 1948; VERLINDE, 1948; WHITNEY and WHITNEY, 1953; INNES, 1949; LAUDER et al., 1954; COFFIN and LIU, 1957; CAMPBELL, 1957; McGRATH, 1960; GORHAM, 1960; BINDRICH, 1962; CORNWELL et al., 1965 a; ARNOLD et al., 1968).

CARRÉ (1905) described distemper as an acute contagious disease in dogs characterized by a diphasic temperature rise, leukopenia, coryza, conjunctivitis, and gastrointestinal and respiratory signs. A small proportion of affected dogs developed nervous manifestations and skin pustules.

LAIDLAW and DUNKIN (1926 a), experimenting with distemper in well-isolated dogs, found a great variation in the severity of clinical signs. They described distemper as an acute febrile disease with fever beginning 3 to 6 days after exposure. The temperature curve was diphasic, the second rise occurred several days after the first. Coryza, vomiting, diarrhea, cough, skin rash, and transient keratitis were seen in some animals. Many dogs recovered. Nervous symptoms were mentioned but not described. Skin pustules, often seen in natural cases, were not found in experimental dogs and were believed to be caused by bacterial complication.

INNES (1953) placed natural cases of dogs in three groups: A systemic infection, a combined systemic and nervous form, and a nervous form alone. The systemic infection included fever; anorexia; cough; serous nasal and ocular discharge, which sometimes became mucopurulent; diarrhea and vomiting; and skin pustules of the abdomen.

COFFIN and LIU (1957) separated 3 clinical forms of distemper in a similar way and related them to the presence of virus in different organs (see Pathogenesis).

LAUDER et al. (1954) postulated 6 different symptoms to be used as criteria for a clinical diagnosis. At least 4 of these symptoms should be present to confirm a diagnosis. The symptoms were: respiratory signs, diarrhea, catarrhal discharge from eyes or nose, hyperkeratosis of foot pads, nervous manifestation, and duration of the disease for 3 weeks or more. This postulation has been questioned by clinicians.

MCGRATH (1960) described the nervous signs associated with distemper in dogs. They were found to be complex and included cranial nerve, meningeal, cerebral, midbrain, cerebellar, vestibular, and spinal cord malfunctions. Single signs suggesting local brain or cord lesions occurred, but more often multiple signs were observed. Cranial nerve signs were described to be rare except for signs resulting from optic nerve damage. Abnormal light reflex and optic placing reactions were seen, occasionally dogs were blind. Tic or flexor spasms of the temporal muscles could be related to lesions of the fifth cranial nerve. Meningeal signs included hyperesthesia, hyperthermia, and cervical rigidity. Cerebral signs were convulsive seizures, incoordination, pacing or propulsion, circling, and psychic changes. Midbrain, cerebellar, vestibular, and medullary signs were characterized by disturbance in gait and posture, including ataxia, asynergy, paresis, torticollis, nystagmus, and others. Hyperkinesia or rhythmic motor movements, usually called chorea, tic, tremor, or myoclonus were common neurologic signs during distemper or as a residual phenomenon.

BREAZILE et al. (1966) found distemper myoclonus to be caused by neuronal damage within one or at most two or three spinal cord segments, by means of segmentation of the spinal cord. It was not reflexly induced, because transaction of dorsal roots did not abolish myoclonus.

CORNWELL et al. (1965 a) found a great variety of clinical signs between and within litters receiving the same strain of virus by contact exposure. The onset of serous conjunctivitis ranged from 5 to 13 days, of catarrhal conjunctivitis from 15 to 41 days, and of purulent conjunctivitis from 17 to 44 days. First cough was noticed 11 to 23 days postexposure, diarrhea 3 to 9 days. Nervous signs were seen in two dogs, beginning 36 and 52 days postexposure. Hyperkeratosis of foot pads in some dogs was noticed 19 days after exposure or later.

A suggested change in the clinical distemper picture occurred in Europe between 1945 and 1948. Hyperkeratosis of the foot pads was becoming a prominent symptom. Persistent tonsillitis and diarrhea was seen in many cases and a high percentage of dogs developed a nervous manifestation of the disease. It was called "hard pad" disease.

MACINTYRE et al. (1948) postulated "hard pad" disease to be different from classical distemper. This problem has been discussed in many publications: COHRS, 1951; FANKHAUSER, 1951; SCHEITLIN et al., 1951; FENNER and SCHINDLER, 1952; MANSI, 1952; LARIN, 1954; and GORHAM, 1960. However, KOPROWSKI et al. (1950), DRÄGER and SCHINDLER (1951), CABASSO and COX (1952), CABASSO (1952), GILLESPIE et al. (1958), and POTEL and BINDRICH (1958) demonstrated the virus involved in "hard pad" disease to be immunologically and serologically identical to the classical distemper virus.

A disease syndrome in middle aged or older dogs named "old dog encephalitis" or subacute diffuse sclerosing encephalomyelitis (CORDY, 1942; VAN BOGAERT and INNES, 1962) has been postulated to be caused by CDV. The disease is characterized by progressive motor and mental deterioration that is ultimately fatal. A panencephalitis with invasion of mononuclear cells, inclusion bodies in glial cells and neurons and some demyelination were the most common pathological lesions. A similarity to human subacute sclerosing panencephalitis has been stated. Recently CD viral antigen has been found with fluorescent antibody in neurons and glial cells in cerebral cortex, thalamus, mesencephalon and medulla of 2 dogs with disseminated panencephalomyelitis. Filamentous microtubules similar to myxovirus nucleocapsids were seen by electron microscopy (LINCOLN, personal communication).

Retention of teeth in dogs as a sequel to CD infection (BODINGBAUER, 1960) is a common observation.

For references to CD in animals other than dogs see Experimental Host Range (p. 29).

2. Mixed Infections with Canine Distemper Virus

a) Bacterial and Mycoplasma

There is general agreement that bacterial organisms play a vital, but secondary role, in respiratory infections associated with field cases of CD (LAIDLAW and DUNKIN, 1926 a; HARDENBERGH, 1925). According to DUNKIN and LAIDLAW (1926 b) purulent conjunctivitis, rhinitis, bronchitis, and bronchopneumonia did not occur in experimental dogs infected with the virus alone and maintained in isolation units.

HSIUNG and STAFSETH (1952) made a comprehensive bacteriologic study of the disease in dogs presented at the veterinary clinic at Michigan State University. Staphylococcus epidermidis was the most prevalent organism in the nasal and conjunctival exudates of dogs during various seasons of the year, irrespective to a diagnosis of canine distemper. Except for Bordetella bronchiseptica which was isolated only from dogs with canine distemper (28.5 per cent) there was little difference in the bacterial flora between dogs with clinical distemper and others without distemper. Other important secondary bacterial invaders in distemper were Micrococcus caseolyticus, Micrococcus aurantiacus, hemolytic streptococci (groups C and D), and nonhemolytic streptococci. Pasteurella tularensis was isolated from dog spleens used for the production of canine distemper vaccine. Experimentally induced tularemia in dogs resembled canine distemper infection.

LAUDER et al. (1954) made anaerobic cultures from the lungs of 70 cases of distemper. No anaerobic bacteria were found in 63 per cent whereas 22 per cent revealed streptococci, 13 per cent Escherichia coli, 8 per cent Proteus vulgaris, and 4 per cent S. epidermidis. In contrast to other reports B. bronchiseptica was not isolated from any of the lungs. These results were comparable to those reported by MACINTYRE et al. (1948). B. bronchiseptica was believed to be the only cause of CD for more than a decade (McGOWAN, 1911). SCHLINGMANN (1932) isolated Bordetella from 81 of 100 dogs with CD.

GUTEKUNST (1957) studied *Mycoplasma* in dogs with and without canine distemper. He found a greater incidence of *Mycoplasma* in dogs with distemper than without. These isolates were nonpathogenic for dogs.

b) Viral

DeMonbreun (1937) inadvertently made the first report of experimental dual infection of dogs with canine distemper and infectious canine hepatitis (ICH) viruses. Unfortunately, his seed virus stock not only contained CDV but, unknown to him, ICHV as well. This is understandable because ICH was not described as a separate entity in dogs until 1948 (Rubarth). DeMonbreun's findings nicely fit into our present knowledge of what constitutes dual infection with these two viruses in the dog. Lewis (1950) found inclusions of both viruses in a natural case of the dog. This is not an unusual finding as many individuals have unreported cases in their files.

GILLESPIE et al. (1952) studied the effects of both viruses given intravenously to experimental dogs maintained in isolation. ICH and CD viruses were both recovered from the blood of dogs given both viruses simultaneously. Approximately 58 per cent of the dogs given ICH only died and 17 per cent with CD only whereas 79 per cent given the mixture died, half on the third day postinoculation. In those dogs given ICHV first followed by CDV 21 days later 89 per cent died. CD inclusion bodies were found in those dogs given CDV only; ICH inclusion bodies in those pups given ICHV only; and inclusion bodies to both viruses in those dogs receiving the mixture of viruses.

Mixed viral infections in the respiratory tract appear to be common. Reovirus (Lou and Wenner, 1963), canine herpesvirus (Motohashi and Tajima, 1966), a parainfluenza virus similar to SV 5, and an adenovirus (Appel and Percy, 1970; Appel et al., 1970) have been found in combination with distemper. Mixed infections frequently occur where CD susceptible dogs are kept in groups (Bjotvedt et al., 1969).

Distemper virus was probably also involved in the "infectious rhinotonsillitis", described by Fontaine et al. (1957), Goret et al. (1959), and Fontaine et al. (1961). Florio et al. (1965) found distemper virus and increasing serum antibody titers against it in dogs with the disease. A second agent has not been ruled out nor confirmed.

HAIG et al. (1956) reported an epizootic of distemper and African horsesickness in 30 of 50 foxhounds. Clinical signs were similar to those commonly seen in CD including nervous signs prior to death. Necropsy showed pulmonary edema, hydrothorax, splenic enlargement, and enteritis. Pulmonary edema and hydrothorax are not associated with CD infection so this suggests that African horsesickness virus played some role in the disease syndrome. African horsesickness virus was isolated from the blood from one fatal case. Neutralizing antibody to African horsesickness virus detected in 19 of the afflicted dogs. CDV was isolated from the brain of one dog which showed nervous signs.

Concurrent infection in ferrets with influenza and distemper viruses did not alter the clinical picture in ferrets (Horsfall and Lennette, 1940). Ferrets given influenza virus only produced high levels of neutralizing antibody and virus was not isolated from their lungs 6 days after infection. In contrast ferrets given both viruses simultaneously produced low levels of influenza-neutralizing antibody and influenza virus was isolated from ferret lungs throughout the course of infection.

Contamination of egg-adapted CDV by avian leukosis virus (PAYNE et al., 1966) did not induce pathological changes in dogs and antibody to several strains of Rous sarcoma virus (RSV) was not made.

DALLDORF (1939) found lymphocytic choriomeningitis (LCM) virus as a contaminant in a serial passage of commercial distemper virus. The effects of CDV and LCM together produced a disease in dogs similar to one caused by CDV alone. DALLDORF recognized the contaminant after study of the disease produced in rhesus monkeys that he originally thought was caused by CDV. A group of three related cases of LCM of unusual severity in individuals preparing canine distemper vaccine was reported by ARMSTRONG (1954).

c) Protozoal

It has been suggested that CDV may activate latent *Toxoplasma* infections in dogs and mink (PRIDHAM and MELCHER, 1958). Dual infections have been observed in dogs by MÖLLER (1962), SIIM et al. (1963), MÖLLER and NIELSEN (1964), and CAPEN and COLE (1966), and in mink by MOMBERG-JØRGENSEN (1965) and PRIDHAM and BELCHER (1958).

Coccidiosis during CD infection appears to be a very common complication in young dogs (BALCON et al., 1967). Distemper infection probably reduces resistance to coccidial infection, and the combined infection appears more severe.

3. Pathology

On gross postmortem inspection very few changes can be seen in cases of uncomplicated distemper in dogs except for a significant reduction in size of the thymus in young dogs, which sometimes appears gelatinous (GIBSON et al., 1965; APPEL, 1969). Interstitial pneumonia and/or catarrhal enteritis may be noticed. Congested meninges may be seen in cases of distemper meningitis and encephalitis. Hyperkeratosis of footpads and nose may be present. Mucopurulent discharges, bronchopneumonias, hemorrhagic enteritis, and skin pustules are probably caused by secondary bacterial infections, which are present in almost all cases of natural distemper. GILLESPIE et al. (1956) observed hemorrhagic enteritis in infant puppies that were kept in isolation.

Histological changes in dogs have been reported frequently (DUNKIN and LAIDLAW, 1926; CORDY, 1942; HURST et al., 1943; MACINTYRE et al., 1948; FANKHAUSER, 1951; POTEL, 1951; SCHEITLIN et al., 1951; COHRS, 1951; LAUDER et al., 1954; GILLESPIE and RICKARD, 1956; CAMPBELL, 1957; INNES and SAUNDERS, 1962; and CORNWELL et al., 1965 a). (For the distribution of inclusion bodies see: Diagnosis, p. 64.) In general, a depletion of lymphocytes was described in lymphatic tissues and swelling and proliferation of reticulum cells so that these tissues appeared loose and edematous in the acute phase. Small lymphocyte depletion was diminished in adrenalectomized CD infected dogs (JACOBY and GRIESEMER, 1970). Regenerative hyperplasia began when the systemic infection subsided. Inclusion bodies were seen in lymphocytes and reticular cells. A diffuse interstitial pneumonia was present with thickening of alveolar walls by fibrous tissue, hyperplasia, and proliferation of alveolar epithelium. Desquamated epithelial cells and macrophages appeared in alveoli. Giant cells were sometimes seen. Inclusion bodies were prominent in bronchial epithelium. Degenerative changes and inclusions were found in the epithelium of stomach and intestine and in the biliary and pancreatic ducts. Transitional epithelium of the urinary tract appeared swollen and hydropic. Urinary bladder and kidney pelvis epithelium had many inclusions. Mild interstitial epididymitis and orchitis were common. MATTHIAS (1957) described degenerative changes in the adrenal gland, mostly cortex. JUBB et al. (1957) described intraocular lesions in cases of distemper. There was a leukocytic infiltration in the ciliary body. Exudative or degenerative changes were seen in retinal ganglion cells, and proliferation in pigment epithelium. Edema produced focal retinal detachments. Ulcerative keratitis sometimes complicated a purulent conjunctivitis.

GIBSON et al. (1965) inoculated 12 gnotobiotic puppies 6 to 9 weeks old, either with virulent Snyder Hill or Lederle strains of CDV. Pups were kept in sterile plastic isolators. The only clinical response to these virulent strains was fever and some decrease in appetite. When puppies were euthanized between 4 and 19 days after intraperitoneal inoculation, the only gross lesion found was a significant size reduction of the thymus. Pathological changes were only observed in lymphatic tissue and in the central nervous system. No lesions were seen in the lungs, skin, or intestine. No inclusion bodies were demonstrated in the conjunctiva, retina, stomach, kidney, or urinary bladder. However, only three puppies were kept for 2 weeks or longer and they had protective antibody titers.

A considerable interest in central nervous lesions in distemper was expressed in many publications (WHITTEM and BLOOD, 1950; WINQUIST, 1950; COHRS, 1951; FANKHAUSER, 1951; SCHEITLIN et al., 1951; POTEL, 1951; FENNER and SCHINDLER, 1952; MANSI, 1952; KRETSCHMAR, 1954; LAUDER et al., 1954; GILLESPIE and RICKARD, 1956; CAMPBELL, 1957; FRAUCHIGER and FANKHAUSER, 1957; McGRATH, 1960; INNES and SAUNDERS, 1962; FISCHER, 1965; GIBSON et al., 1965; PECKHAM, 1967). A special stimulus was the attempt to differentiate between lesions in classical distemper and "hard pad" disease. Because a general agreement had been achieved that no basic difference existed between the two diseases, no difference will be made in the discussion of distemper encephalitis.

Histopathological lesions ranged from minimal inflammation (CORDY, 1942; LAUDER et al., 1954; GIBSON et al., 1965) to severe disseminated meningoencephalomyelitis with demyelination (INNES and SAUNDERS, 1962). Distemper virus had an affinity for both the white and the gray matter in brain and spinal cord and lesions occurred in any part of the central nervous system. Eosinophilic inclusion bodies have been demonstrated in the different types of glial cells, in neurons, ependymal, and meningeal cells. Structures most consistently affected were the cerebellar peduncles, medulla, pons, midbrain, basal ganglia, cerebral cortex, optic tracts, and meninges. Tissue around the fourth ventricle appeared to be a predelective site (INNES and SAUNDERS, 1962).

Meningitis was almost constantly present with cellular changes in the pia-arachnoid region. Cellular infiltrate consisted mainly of lymphocytes, plasma cells, and undifferentiated mononuclear cells. Swelling and desquamation of meningeal cells and an increase in meningeal macrophages could be seen together with hypertrophy and hyperplasia of perivascular cells (CAMPBELL, 1957).

Vascular changes included dilated and hyperemic capillaries and venules of brain, spinal cord, and leptomeninges. Edema with single lymphocytes and plasma cells occurred in Virchow-Robin spaces, meninges, choroid plexus, and subependymal tissues (COHRS, 1951). Perivascular hemorrhages were seen occasionally. Perivascular "cuffing" occurred in 28 of 50 dogs studied by CAMPBELL (1957),

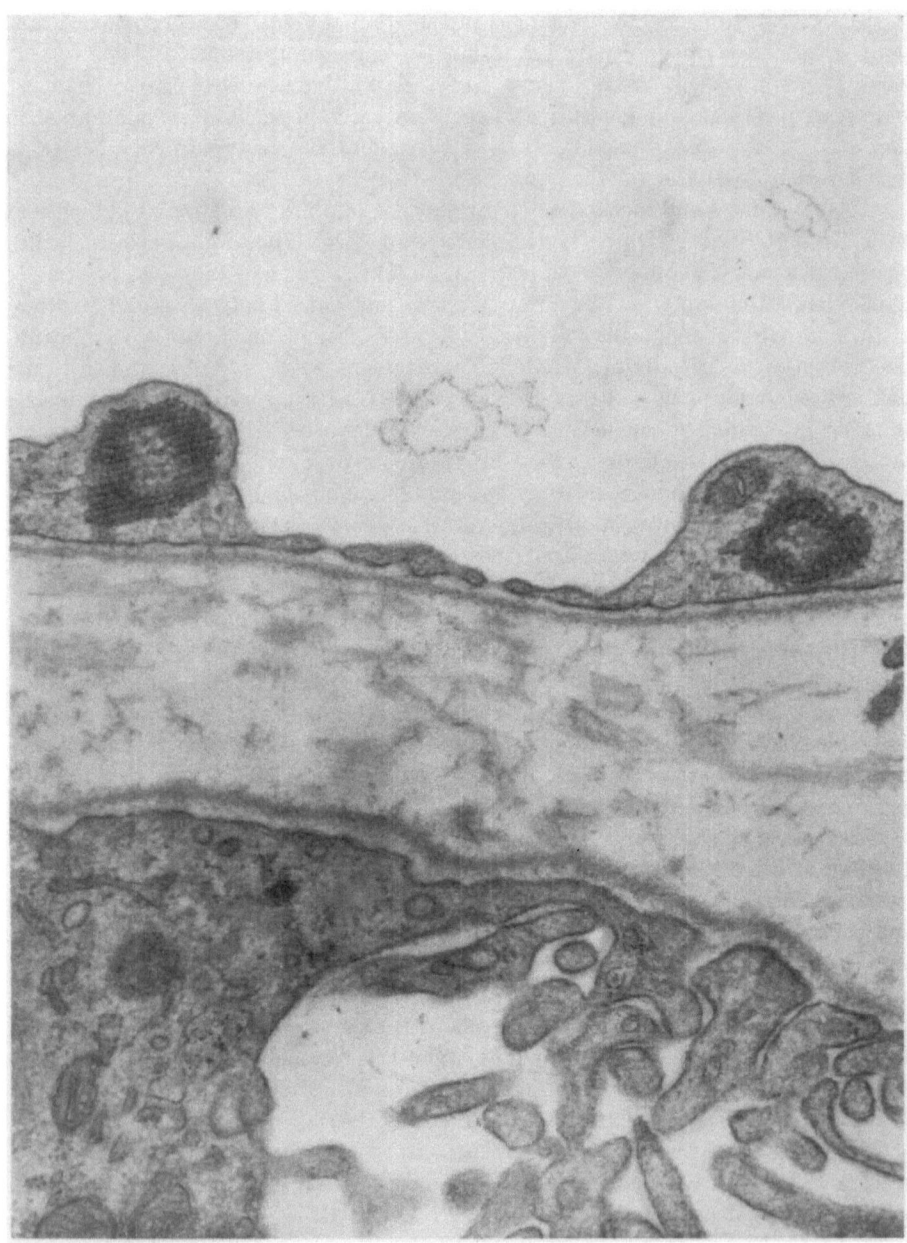

Fig. 23. Canine distemper nucleocapsid-like structures in plexus capillaries of a dog with distemper encephalitis (× 60,000). Courtesy of N. DEUTSCHLÄNDER, University of Munich, Germany

consisting of mostly lymphocytes and some plasma cells. Ependymal changes were most apparent in the third and fourth ventricle and consisted of edema, vacuolation, loss of cilia, and some destruction of ependymal cells (CAMPBELL, 1957).

By electron microscopy, crystal-like structures similar to CD nucleocapsids

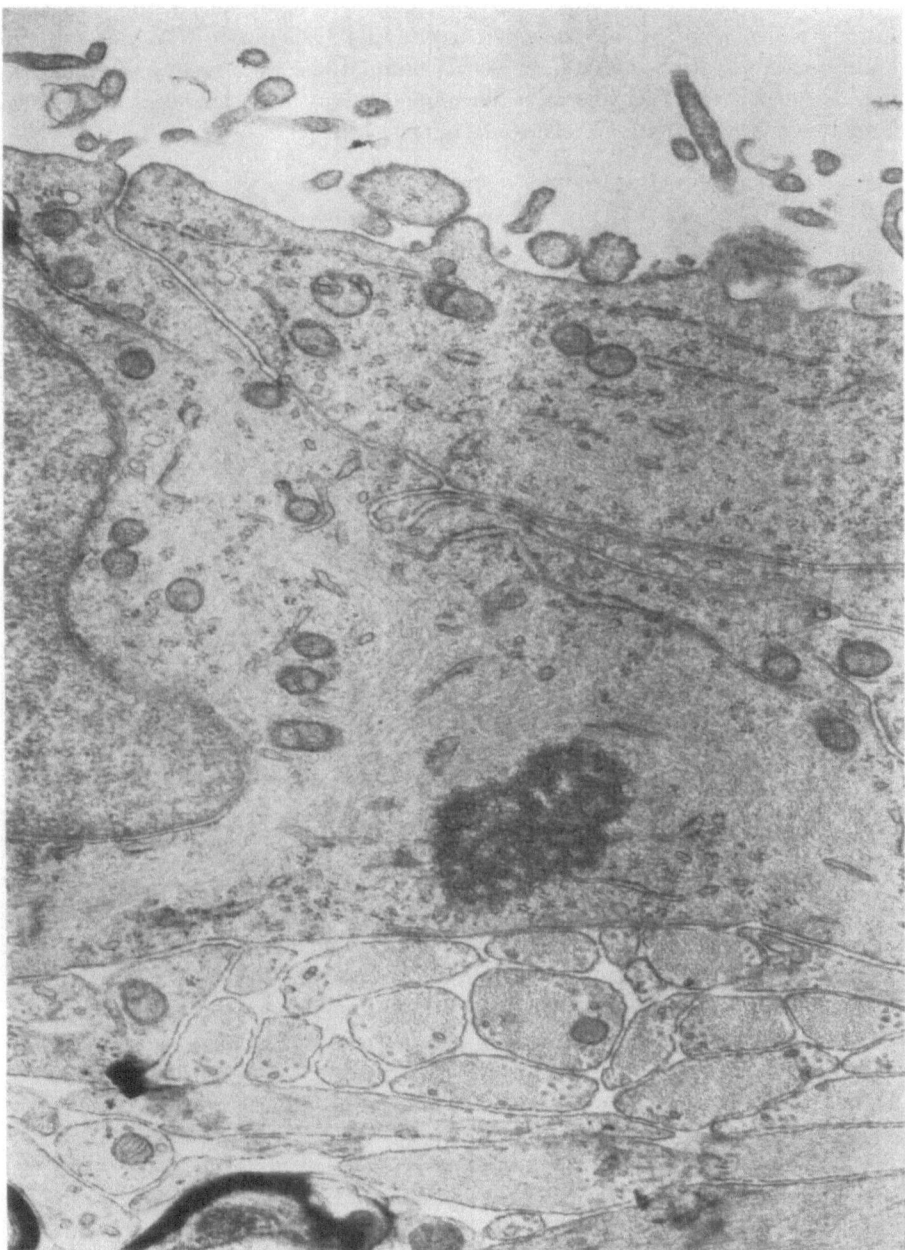

Fig. 24. Canine distemper nucleocapsid-like structures in ependymal cells of a dog with distemper encephalitis (× 42,000). Courtesy of N. DEUTSCHLÄNDER, University of Munich, Germany

were seen in the cytoplasm of endothelial and adventitial cells of meningeal veins and arteries, in the endothelium of cortical and plexus capillaries (Fig. 23), in mononuclear cells within the lumen of blood vessels, in histiocytes and macrophages within the subarachnoid space, in reactive microglia cells, and in ependymal cells (Fig. 24) (BLINZINGER and DEUTSCHLÄNDER, 1969).

Neuroglial changes included microglia, oligodendroglia, and astrocytes. Glial foci developed and, besides inclusion bodies (see: Diagnosis, p. 64), swelling of cytoplasm and nuclei was noticed. Cell accumulations were mostly seen in myelinated zones. With demyelination developing many neuroglial cells became enlarged and formed "Gitter" cells (CAMPBELL, 1957).

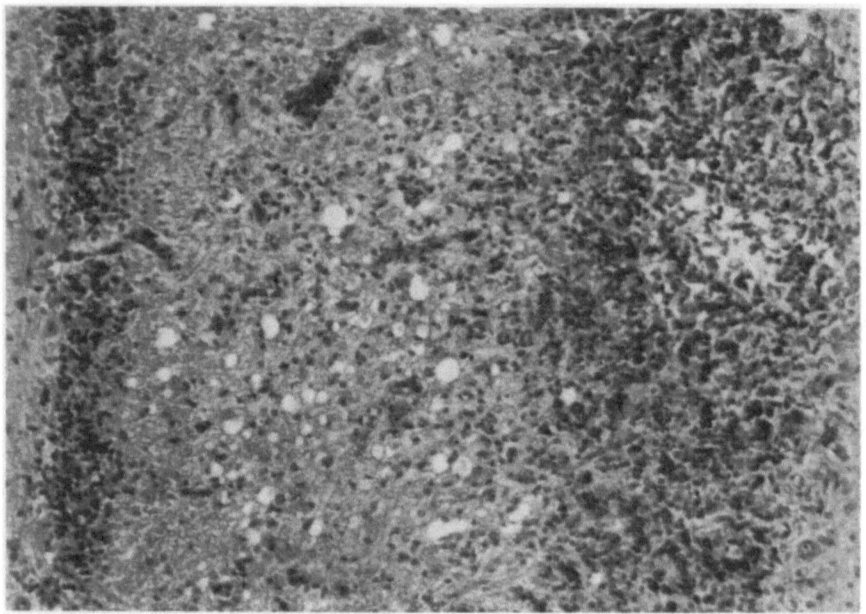

Fig. 25. Demyelination and gliosis in cerebellar folia of a dog with canine distemper. H and E stain (× 80). Courtesy of A. de LAHUNTA, New York State Veterinary College

Neuronal degeneration was found by most authors. There was much contradiction in the literature regarding the occurrence of inclusion bodies in neurons. Viral antigen was demonstrated in neurons (LIU and COFFIN, 1957; APPEL, 1969).

Demyelination (Fig. 25) is often a prominent feature of dogs with CD nervous manifestations. GILLESPIE and RICKARD (1956) found demyelination in dogs with epileptiform convulsions at 22 days but not in dogs with similar signs 16 days or less after inoculation with the Snyder Hill strain. CAMPBELL (1957) observed demyelination in 25 of 50 dogs. Cerebellar folia and peduncles appeared to be more affected than other areas in the brain. In early stages white matter was rarefied (status cribrosus or spongiosus) and contained few "Gitter" cells. In severe cases, massive breakdown of myelin and axis cylinders occurred with dense glial hyperplasia and infiltration. "Gitter" cells were abundant. Distemper demyelination has been discussed in many publications (GORHAM, 1960, INNES and SAUNDERS, 1962; FRAUCHIGER and FANKHAUSER, 1969).

Neurological manifestations of CD, including demyelination, have caused considerable speculation about its pathogenesis (TREVAN, 1953) because demyelinating human diseases are still unsolved problems. For a long period the autoimmune concept has been favored for explaining human demyelinating diseases. Similarities with experimental allergic encephalomyelitis induced by a brain basic protein (PATERSON, 1966) were remarkable. Cellular or humoral brain antibody in the presence of complement (BORNSTEIN and RAINE, 1970) induced demyelination in various experimental animals. ALVORD et al. (1968) attempted to react post-distemper dog sera with brain proteins, but results were elusive. The isolation of measles virus or a measles-like virus from patients with subacute sclerosing panencephalitis (HORTA-BARBOSA et al., 1969) did not rule out the autoimmune concept. However, a direct virus effect on oligodendroglia cells, which produce myelin, has to be considered. STORTS et al. (1968) induced demyelination in brain explants with CD virus (cf. p. 17).

Pathological changes in ferrets and mink have been described by CROOK and McNUTT (1959) and SAWADA (1965). Lesions were similar to those in dogs. They appeared more slowly in mink than in ferrets, and mink showed more ability than ferrets to regenerate lymphoid tissue. This evidence may account for the difference in mortality rates of ferrets and of mink. Pathology of CD in experimental animals has been referred to in that section.

4. Diagnosis

The general picture of canine distemper has changed since attenuated virus vaccines and antibiotics are commonly used. Less acute cases are seen and in many dogs pathognomonic symptoms (LAUDER et al., 1954) are absent.

On postmortem inspection, uncomplicated distemper reveals very little gross changes except a considerable reduction in size of the thymus (GIBSON et al., 1965). This observation is nonspecific. It can be observed after any prolonged stress condition. Consequently, laboratory tests are required for the diagnosis of canine distemper.

a) Ferret Inoculation

For a long time, secretions or tissue suspensions from infected dogs were inoculated into susceptible ferrets (LAIDLAW and DUNKIN, 1926; GREEN, 1939; McINTYRE et al., 1948; CROOK et al., 1958). When distemper virus was present in the inoculum, ferrets died from distemper between 10 to 14 days after inoculation. When the effect could be neutralized by pretreating the inoculum with specific antibody, the diagnosis was confirmed. Some investigators found a prolonged incubation period in ferrets (LARIN, 1954; RECULARD and GUILLON, 1967), however, on a serological basis no difference could be demonstrated.

b) Virus Isolation in Tissue Culture

More recently, tissue culture systems have been employed for the isolation of virulent distemper virus. VANTSIS (1959) found ferret kidney cell cultures to be susceptible for virulent virus. Giant cell formation after several days of infection indicated the presence of distemper virus. CORNWELL et al. (1965 b) used this technique for virus isolation in their experimental work with distemper. However, they found ferret kidney cell cultures less sensitive than the living ferret for the detection of distemper virus. BUSSEL and KARZON (1965 a) reported similar observations. APPEL and JONES (1967) used dog alveolar macrophage cultures for distemper virus propagation. Giant cells in these cultures appeared from 2 to 5 days postinoculation. Virus was isolated from nasal, oral, conjunctival, and fecal swabs and from cerebrospinal fluid from dogs with acute distemper. When cells were cultured from bronchial washings of euthanized dogs with systemic distemper, giant cells appeared between 1 and 16 hours after culturing. Overlays on dog kidney cell or Vero cell monolayer cultures of buffy coat cells from dogs with acute CD resulted in CDV isolation (APPEL, unpublished).

c) Complement Fixation Test

LAIDLAW and DUNKIN (1931) first employed the complement fixation test in distemper to estimate the viral content of various tissues. This test has been used extensively later in diagnosis and research to demonstrate viral antigen in a wide variety of tissues, especially by German investigators: MITSCHERLICH (1938), DEDIÉ (1951), DEDIÉ and KLAPÖTKE (1951, 1952), DRÄGER and SCHINDLER (1951), BINDRICH (1954). Tissues used for viral antigen included: spleen, lymph nodes, bone marrow, thymus, brain, lung, liver, kidneys, thyroid, salivary glands, pancreas, urine, and cerebrospinal fluid.

d) Inclusion Bodies

Intracytoplasmic and, less frequently, intranuclear eosinophilic inclusion bodies are considered pathognomonic for distemper. They were found in epithelial cells, reticulum cells, leukocytes, glial cells, and neurons. Numerous reports appeared on inclusion bodies in distemper diagnosis. STANDFUSS (1908) and LENTZ (1909) described distemper inclusions in neurons and glial cells to differentiate them from Negri bodies. BROADHURST et al. (1938), Goss et al. (1948), LINDGREN (1951), GUARDA and DOTTA (1959), CELLO et al. (1959), DONOVAN and OTT (1960), ERNÖ (1963, 1964), CORNWELL et al. (1965 a), SCHÖBEL (1968), SCHRÖDER et al. (1968), and others attempted distemper diagnosis in the living dog by staining swab and smear preparations from mucous membranes. Samples from conjunctiva, nasal mucosa, tongue, vagina, prepuce, and urethra were found to contain inclusion bodies but not in all CD cases that were examined. DONOVAN and OTT (1960) found distemper inclusion bodies in epithelial smears made from the conjunctiva, vagina, prepuce, and urethra between 11 and 16 days following vaccination with ferret or egg-adapted modified live distemper virus. These findings were not confirmed by other investigators (SCHÖBEL, 1968). CELLO et al. (1959) found cytoplasmic inclusions in circulating neutrophils, which persisted for several months. This observation was not confirmed (CORNWELL et al., 1965 a).

Inclusion bodies in conjunctival cells were found by CELLO et al. (1959) in 10 of 16, by GUARDA (1959) in 25 of 30, by ERNO (1964) in 30 of 100, by SCHRÖDER et al. (1968) in 83 of 114, and by SCHÖBEL (1968) in only 18 of 117 dogs with clinical distemper. CORNWELL et al. (1965 a) found inclusions in contact dogs only between 11 and 18 days after exposure.

GREEN and EVANS (1939), SJOLTE (1947), LINDGREN (1951), LAUDER et al. (1954), CAMPBELL et al. (1955), ERNO (1964), FISCHER (1965 a), GIBSON et al. (1965)

and others demonstrated distemper inclusions in paraffin sections, using various stains. GREEN and EVANS (1939) summarized the literature on distemper inclusions. They found them in epithelium of various organs and lymphocytes but not in vascular endothelium. SJOLTE (1947) examined 28 dogs and found inclusion bodies in 70 per cent of them. LINDGREN (1951) took trachea and urinary bladder smears from 60 distemper dogs and found inclusions in 66 per cent. LAUDER et al. (1954) found distemper inclusions in 44 of 50 examined cases or 88 per cent. The distribution of inclusions in different tissues was given: lung 78 per cent, mediastinal lymph node 46 per cent, exocrine cells of pancreas 50 per cent, duodenum 14 per cent, spleen 39 per cent, kidney 52 per cent, urinary bladder 53 per cent, foot pads 40 per cent, and central nervous system 68 per cent. Cytoplasmic inclusions may persist for 5 or 6 weeks in the lymphatic system and in the urinary tract. Some inclusions persisted even longer in brain and lung. Few inclusions were seen in the early phase of the disease. Similar findings were observed by other investigators.

v. MICKWITZ and SCHRÖDER (1968) observed viral antigen in inclusions with fluorescent antibody, but H & E stained inclusions persisted longer than viral antigen in dogs that recovered from distemper. On the other hand, not all viral antigen seen in tissues with fluorescent antibody was observed as inclusion bodies by H & E stain. They found viral antigen but not inclusion bodies in 12 per cent of their examined tissues. They considered the fluorescent technique superior to the finding of inclusion bodies for diagnosis.

e) Fluorescent-Antibody Test

MOULTON and BROWN (1954) first applied the fluorescent antibody (FA) technique for distemper diagnosis. They found viral antigen in smear preparations from urinary bladders of infected dogs. The effect could partially be blocked with unlabelled distemper antiserum. MOULTON (1956) reported viral antigen in astrocytes of brain white matter during the process of demyelination in distemper infected dogs. LIU and COFFIN (1957) made extensive FA studies on the distribution of viral antigen in distemper infected ferrets and dogs (see: Pathogenesis, p. 34). They found conjunctival smears and organ imprints from dogs with acute distemper suitable for diagnosis. CELLO et al. (1959) were able to find viral antigen in neutrophil granulocytes to persist in recovered dogs. This observation has not been confirmed. MAESTRONE (1963) found viral antigen in cells that had been fixed with formalin. However, a special tissue treatment was required.

More recently several reports were made on the use of FA for distemper diagnosis (MATTHIAS, 1966; BAUMANN, 1967; FAIRCHILD et al., 1967, 1971; SCHRÖDER et al., 1968; MOTOHASHI et al., 1969). APPEL (1969) labelled blood leukocyte preparations (Fig. 26), conjunctival smears (Fig. 27), and cerebrospinal fluid cells of aerosol exposed specific pathogen-free dogs with FA in addition to tissue sections (see: Pathogenesis, p. 37). Results were related to presence of serum neutralizing antibody (Figs. 28, 29). Viral antigen in buffy coat cells was first noted 2 days PI in some dogs, it was present in all dogs 5 days PI. In dogs that developed measurable neutralizing antibody 8 or 9 days PI, no more viral antigen could be detected. In dogs that failed to produce a protective titer of antibody, buffy coat cells were seen to contain viral antigen until dogs died from acute

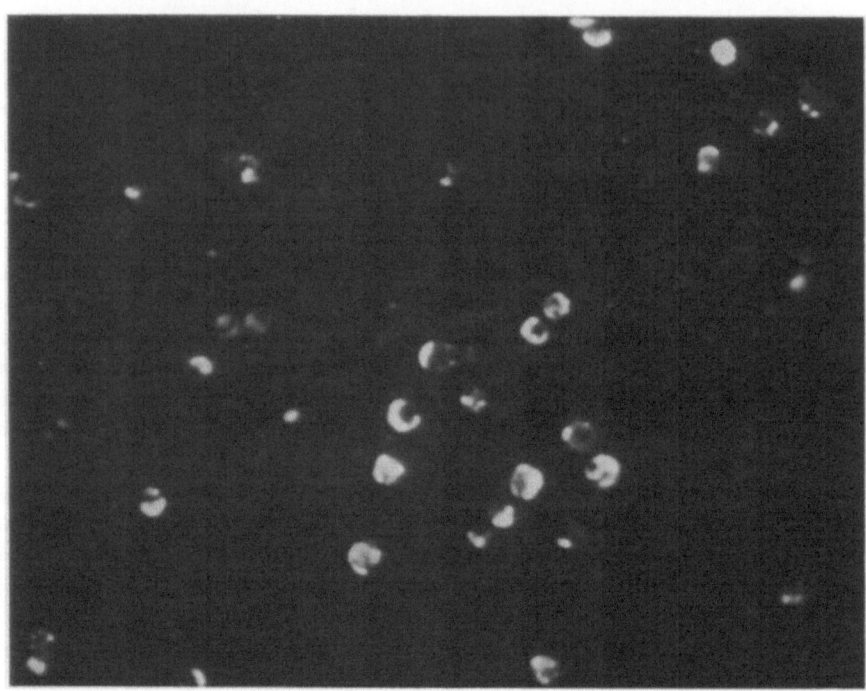

Fig. 26. Fluorescent mononuclear cells in blood leukocyte preparation of dog 7 days after it was exposed to aerosol of canine distemper virus (× 250). Reprinted with permission from: APPEL, M. J. G.: Amer. J. vet. Res. **30**, 1167 (1969)

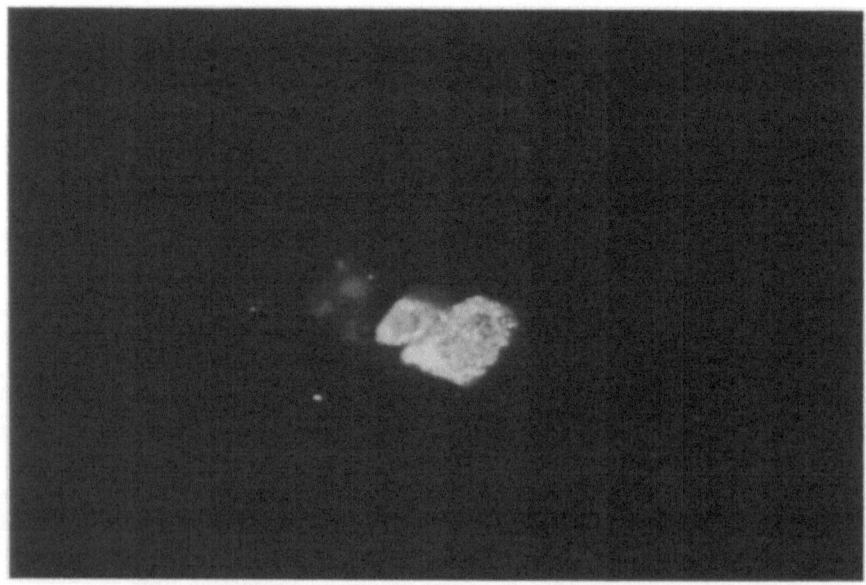

Fig. 27. Fluorescent granules in cells of a conjunctival smear from a dog with canine distemper without neutralizing antibody (× 250). Reprinted with permission from: APPEL, M. J. G.: Amer. J. vet. Res. **30**, 1167 (1969)

distemper 3 to 4 weeks PI. Viral antigen in conjunctival cells appeared only 7 days PI. It persisted in dogs with low antibody titers and was not seen after serum antibody levels became protective for dogs. Cells from cerebrospinal fluid contained viral antigen only 11 or more days after exposure in dogs that failed to develop

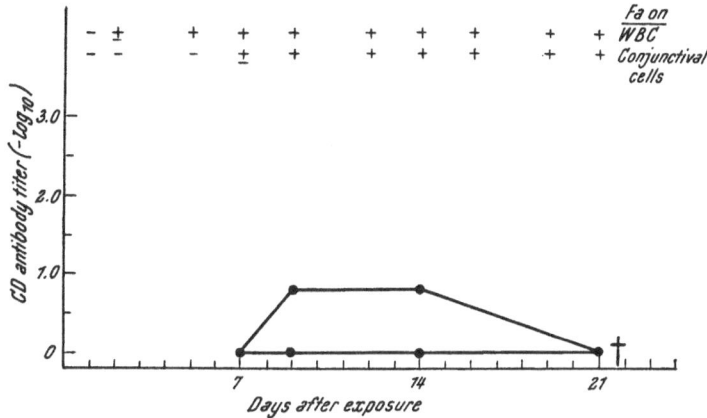

Fig. 28. Persistence of canine distemper (CD) virus and formation of antibodies in 6 dogs which were exposed to aerosol of CD virus and which died. Reprinted with permission from: APPEL, M. J. G.: Amer. J. vet. Res. **30**, 1167 (1969)

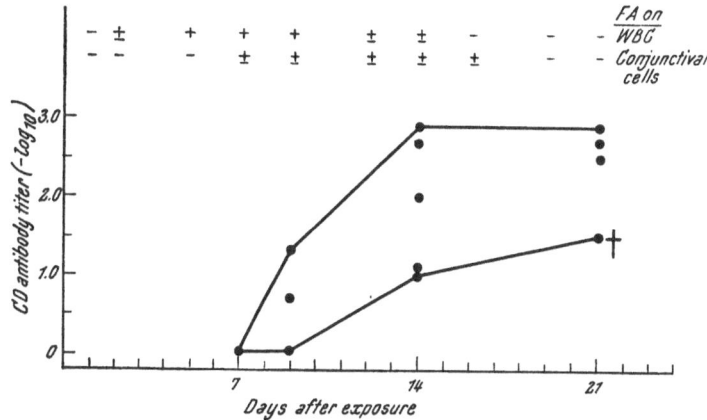

Fig. 29. Persistence of canine distemper (CD) virus and formation of antibodies in 5 dogs which were exposed to aerosol of CD virus and which survived, except for 1 dog which died. Reprinted with permission from: APPEL, M. J. G.: Amer. J. vet. Res. **30**, 1167 (1969)

protective serum antibody titers. Samples taken from field dogs with natural distemper exposure (APPEL, 1970) revealed a similar inverse relationship between presence of viral antigen and antibody. When serum antibody titers were 1 : 100 or greater viral antigen could not be seen in buffy coat of conjunctival cells, but it was seen in frozen sections prepared from foot pad biopsies of some cases. Similar results were obtained by FAIRCHILD (1967, 1971) and MOTOMISHI et al. (1969). SCHRÖDER et al. (1968) found conjunctival smears from 70 of 148 distemper dogs positive with FA.

BAUMANN (1967) examined impression smears and frozen sections from 75 dogs with natural distemper. The tissues tested in most cases were from several parts of the brain, lungs, stomach, kidney, pelvis, and urinary bladder. She found impression smears suitable for distemper diagnosis. Viral antigen could be seen in one or more tissues of 74 dogs. In 81 per cent of dogs with encephalitic signs viral antigen was found in brain cells, while in 70 per cent it was seen in cells from other organs. In dogs with catarrhal distemper the results were reversed: 70 per cent of the dogs had viral antigen in brain cells, while 86 per cent had it in cells from other organs.

v. MICKWITZ and SCHRÖDER (1968) compared H & E staining for inclusion bodies with FA for distemper diagnosis in 23 dogs with clinical distemper, which either died or were euthanized. The dogs' ages ranged from 7 weeks to 11 years, duration of illness from 2 days to 6 weeks. In summary, 12.2 per cent more tissue impressions contained viral antigen than inclusion bodies in H & E sections. The authors recommended FA staining of impression smears from lung, stomach, duodenum, urinary bladder, and brain for distemper diagnosis.

f) Serum Proteins

A decrease in the serum albumin fraction and an increase in the alpha 2 fraction during initial and advanced stages of CD in dogs have been reported (MEBUS and COLES, 1965; SNOW et al., 1966). However, these changes are not specific for CD. Significant changes in serum transaminase activity were found by MARJANOVIC (1969) but not by SNOW et al. (1966).

g) Cerebrospinal Fluid

Besides a nonspecific inflammatory increase in protein and cells in cerebrospinal fluid (CSF) of dogs with CD encephalitis (INNES and SAUNDERS, 1962), a more selective increase in gamma globulin concentrations with presence of IgM and high concentrations of IgG in CSF was reported by CUTLER and AVERILL (1969). Specific CDV neutralizing antibody was only found in CSF of dogs with a subacute form of CD encephalitis, but not in dogs that were either vaccinated, recovered early from CD infection, or died from acute CD infection (APPEL, 1969, 1970).

Increased transaminase activity in CSF was reported by MARJANOVIC (1969).

E. Prevention

1. Active Immunization

Active Immunity against CD in dogs and other susceptible species can be achieved by the use of various types of vaccines. Active immunization has been practiced since PUNTONI (1923) and LAIDLAW and DUNKIN (1928 b, c) and it became very successful after live attenuated vaccines became available (CABASSO et al., 1951; HAIG, 1956; ROCKBORN, 1960). Recommendations and guidelines for CD immunization were summarized in a symposium on canine distemper immunization (GILLESPIE et al., 1966).

a) Inactivated Virus Vaccines

With the introduction of modified live virus vaccines and their wide acceptance by the veterinary profession, the inactivated virus vaccines for CD prophylaxis have assumed less importance. Until 1950, the inactivated virus vaccines were used primarily for immunization of dogs. In 1964, twenty-four per cent of all CD vaccines produced in the United States were still inactivated (TAMOGLIA, 1966).

PUNTONI (1923) vaccinated dogs successfully with formalin-inactivated CDV infected dog brain tissue. LAIDLAW and DUNKIN (1928 b) produced formalin-inactivated virus vaccine from infected ferret tissues that protected ferrets 7 days after injection but not after 4 days. The best protection was afforded after 10 and 14 days between vaccination and challenge. Approximately 75 per cent of these ferrets resisted challenge. They also reported that vaccine prepared from dog tissues had little value in ferrets even when multiple inoculations were given. In addition, inactivated ferret origin vaccine was successful in dogs only after multiple injections were administered. LAIDLAW (1930) postulated that antibody response to the virus might be overshadowed by host response to the heterologous tissue. These investigators felt that a series of injections with inactivated virus vaccine did not confer a long lasting immunity comparable to natural disease. Consequently, they recommended that the series of inactivated virus vaccine injections be followed with an injection of virulent virus to assure lasting and maximal protection. This was not without danger because occasional dogs vaccinated by this procedure developed disease and some died. However, this procedure still seems to be best for the production of hyperimmune serum.

Repeated vaccination with formalin-inactivated virus vaccine plus an adjuvant was recommended by OTT et al. (1959), who found resistance to challenge with virulent CD virus in ferrets one week after vaccination; 78 per cent of the challenged ferrets survived. After injection of formalin- inactivated virus suspension, little or no neutralizing antibody was formed in dogs (GILLESPIE, 1965). When 2 or 3 injections were given, neutralizing antibody titers in dogs reached levels up to 1 : 100. The half-life of this antibody was approximately 15 days and little or no antibody was detected 3 months after the last injection. Dogs challenged at this time with virulent Snyder Hill virus showed little or no clinical disease; however, virus replication was reflected by a sharp rise in antibody titer within 7 days after challenge. Dogs reacted the same way when challenged 2 weeks after one injection of inactivated vaccine. When egg-adapted virus was inoculated 2 weeks after 1, 2, or 3 bi-weekly injections of inactivated virus, increase in antibody titers following virus replication depended upon initial serum antibody titers. Inactivated virus injections in some cases did interfere with the immunizing effect of live virus vaccine.

In summary, virulent virus replicates in dogs or ferrets in most cases when infected after vaccination with inactivated virus. Under normal conditions, a secondary type antibody response blocks clinical disease. If, however, stress or secondary infections complicate this process, clinical disease and death can occur.

b) Live Virus Vaccines

A ferret-passaged CDV vaccine was the first live CD virus vaccine produced for dogs and it has been widely used by veterinarians (WATSON, 1939; GREEN,

1939; GREEN and SWALE, 1939; BODIN, 1947; SMITH, 1958). However, virulence of this virus was only partially reduced and clinical signs often occurred in dogs after vaccination.

The propagation of CDV in the hen's embryonated egg by HAIG (1948) and CABASSO and COX (1949) and its subsequent attenuation through serial passage ultimately made available an excellent vaccine for the immunization of various hosts susceptible to CD. The literature about immunization with avianized CD vaccine was reviewed in detail by HAIG (1956).

The minimum number of egg infectious doses (EID_{50}) of egg-adapted virus required to start replication and immunization in various hosts has been studied carefully. HAIG (1956) concluded that any suspension capable of producing well-defined lesions on the CAM would confer immunity in ferrets and dogs. OTT et al. (1957) found ferrets more susceptible than dogs and required 0.7 log less virus than dogs for production of immunity. BURGHER et al. (1958) found between 64 to 250 EID_{50} of the Lederle avianized strain necessary to produce immunity in the dog. CABASSO et al. (1959) observed that CAM was less sensitive than the ferret for the detection of avianized virus. According to the probit analysis method, two biological units were required to immunize ferrets, but 32 units to immunize mink (SVEHAG and GORHAM, 1962).

Multiplication of egg-adapted virus in the vaccinated host has been found in dogs, ferrets, mink, and foxes (GORHAM, 1957 b). Maximum virus titers in ferrets appeared in spleen and lungs 6 to 9 days after vaccination. Virus was no longer detectable 18 days after vaccination. Vaccine virus or leukopenia were not found in dogs 3 weeks after vaccination (DRÄGER et al., 1956). Spread of egg-adapted virus from dog to dog did not occur (GILLESPIE, 1968). Contact dogs did not develop immunity.

In contrast to virulent virus, egg-adapted virus in dogs did not seem to infect surface epithelium in dogs and replication seemed to be restricted to lymphatic tissues. Dogs on a folic acid deficient diet and treated with Methotrexate had no measurable neutralizing antibody 4 weeks after vaccination with the Lederle strain and CDV was isolated from these dogs from lymphatic tissues only (SHEFFY and APPEL, unpublished). The Wisconsin FXNO strain did not cross the placental barrier in pregnant mink and ferrets (HAGEN et al., 1970). However, this strain reverted to virulence after serial passage in ferrets (GORHAM, personal communication).

Egg-adapted vaccine virus induced resistance in CD susceptible species against challenge with virulent virus, commencing a few days after vaccination. The rapid development of resistance following inoculation of attenuated CDV has been suggested to be interference. Resistance appeared several days before neutralizing antibody could be found in serum. Ferrets inoculated parenterally with egg-adapted CDV 2 or more days before intraperitoneal injection of virulent virus did not develop CD (BAKER et al., 1952; CABASSO et al., 1953 a; GORHAM et al., 1954 a). The quantity of vaccine virus given appeared to be important. Nebulization for a few minutes of egg-adapted virus protected ferrets only 5 days later (GORHAM et al., 1954 a). If the period of nebulization was increased to one hour using identical equipment and virus, resistance was demonstrable in 6 hours (MORRIS et al., 1954). Simultaneous infection of egg-adapted and virulent virus protected ferrets if the ratio of virus was 100 : 1. By increasing the ratio 10,000 : 1 some protection was noted when virulent virus preceded the egg-adapted virus by 24 hours (BURGER and GORHAM, 1964). These ratios have little practical value. Vaccination of dogs after exposure to virulent virus had no effect on the course of the disease (FARRELL et al., 1958; GORHAM, 1960).

When neutralizing antibody appeared in dogs 6 or more days after vaccination and these dogs were challenged with virulent virus, virus multiplication did not seem to occur. Challenge virus has never been isolated from such dogs and an increase in serum antibody titer rarely occurred after challenge. Immunity in most dogs after vaccination was long lasting; however, there were exceptions (ROBSON et al., 1959; KEEBLE, 1962). Duration of immunity has been already discussed (cf. p. 44).

Tissue culture-adapted CD virus vaccines have been used more recently with similar success. Egg-adapted virus has been further adapted to chick embryo fibroblast (CEF) cultures (CABASSO et al., 1959) and virulent virus has been adapted to primary dog kidney (DK) cell cultures (ROCKBORN, 1960) with subsequent vaccine production. A large number of adaptations have been made since, which have been already discussed (cf. p. 18). Tissue culture-adapted CDV vaccines generally are considered to be as effective as egg-adapted CDV vaccines in CD susceptible species and onset and duration of induced resistance and immunity appears to be similar. The immunizing effect for dogs should be tested in dogs, not in ferrets (ROCKBORN et al., 1965).

c) Heterotypic Virus Vaccines

Measles virus (MV) (WARREN et al., 1960; GILLESPIE and KARZON, 1960; MOURA and WARREN, 1961) and rinderpest virus (RV) (POLDING and SIMPSON, 1957) protect dogs against disease when infected later with CDV (see: Immunological Relationship between CDV, MV and RV, p. 48). These original findings have been confirmed in many studies with MV (SLATER and MURDOCK, 1963; BAKER, 1963, 1970; DELAY et al., 1965; ROBERTS, 1965; BAKER et al., 1966; MEBUS and COLES, 1966; ACKERMANN and SIEBEL, 1968; McMANUS, 1968; PRYDIE, 1968; ACKERMANN, 1970; BITTLE, 1970; GALE, 1970; SLATER, 1970). The protection was of particular interest since CD maternal antibody in pups did not interfere with the immunizing effect of MV. In dogs fully susceptible to CDV, the heterotypic MV vaccination had no advantage over attenuated CDV vaccines, since MV only protected dogs from CD disease but not from infection (MEBUS and COLES, 1966; ACKERMANN, 1970; BAKER, 1970; BITTLE, 1970). However, in pups with CD maternal antibody, CDV vaccines did not stimulate active immunity and MV, therefore, was indicated as a heterotypic vaccine (BAKER, 1963, 1966).

The mode of MV induced CD protection has been debated. Some authors favored, without proof, an interferon or interference reaction since protection occurred within a few days (SLATER and MURDOCK, 1963; PEACOCK, 1966). The better explanation appears to be an *anamnestic* MV and CDV antibody response in dogs challenged with CDV after MV inoculation (DELAY et al., 1965; ROBERTS, 1965). The anamnestic response was still found 6 months after MV inoculation (WARREN et al., 1960). BAKER et al. (1968, 1970) found CD serum antibody in MV infected dogs 6 days and in control dogs only 8 or 9 days after CD challenge. In MV vaccinated dogs, less CD virus after challenge was found in spleen tissue than in control dogs and virus was found 6 days after challenge (BAKER, unpublished) in contrast to control dogs that had virus for longer periods. This concept has been strengthened by SLATER (1970) who blocked the protecting effect of MV with immuno-suppressing agents.

It is not definitely known whether measles virus multiplied in dogs. Several isolation attempts of vaccine strains have been unsuccessful (MOURA and WARREN, 1961; ROBERTS, 1965; MEBUS and COLES, 1966). Virus did not spread from dog to dog (GALE, 1970). Measles antibody levels in dogs were related to dose of inoculation similar to an inactivated virus response (SLATER and MURDOCK, 1963; PRYDIE, 1968). Protection against CD challenge was related to MV antibody levels (BITTLE, 1970). A minimum of 10,000 $TCID_{50}$ of MV were required to protect dogs successfully against CD, while only 1,000 $TCID_{50}$ were required for human vaccination. However, formalized MV did not protect dogs (SLATER and MURDOCK, 1963). It must be assumed that low grade multiplication of MV in dogs occurred. Blood from measles patients inoculated into dogs produced a febrile response and catarrhal signs. Serial passages in dogs produced similar signs (BARDACH et al., 1947; RIAZANTSEVA, 1956).

There appear to be a few pitfalls in the use of MV as heterotypic vaccine with CD maternal antibody. Most experiments have been made in 6 week old or older dogs. However, vaccination was recommended for 3 to 4 week old pups and they were not always protected (BITTLE, 1970; GALE, 1970), although high levels of CD maternal antibody did not interfere with MV vaccination (BAKER et al., 1966). The age factor was tested by BAKER (unpublished) by MV inoculation of 3 week old pups. These pups were challenged with virulent CD virus when 10 weeks old. No age difference was found.

Maternal MV antibody may interfere with MV vaccination of pups (BITTLE, 1970). Revaccination with CD vaccine of dogs vaccinated with MV may cause the rise of both CDV and MV antibody (ROBERTS, 1965). BAKER (unpublished) found no interfering effect of maternal MV antibody 2 years after the initial MV inoculation. Only one-third of dams vaccinated as pups with MV passed maternal MV antibody to the first litter and only if the first litter was whelped within the first year.

In summary, dogs inoculated with large doses of MV usually produce homologous antibody only. When challenged with CDV later, CDV growth is restricted and an anamnestic CD antibody response protects dog against clinical distemper. The only indication for MV vaccination is in young pups with maternal CDV antibody.

2. Passive Immunization

Passive immunization against CDV has been used mostly before reliable attenuated CDV vaccines became available. The first investigators who prepared an antiserum of canine origin for the protection of dogs against CD were LOCKHART et al. (1925). They hyperimmunized immune dogs by injections of blood from CD infected dogs which were eliciting a febrile reaction. In time, this product was approved for use by the United States Department of Agriculture. It was used primarily by the simultaneous injection of antiserum and a dose of virulent virus calculated to produce CD in control animals. Using susceptible dogs, LAIDLAW and DUNKIN (1931) showed that hyperimmune CD antisera varied widely in potency. Despite extensive efforts, they were unable to develop a quick and reliable method to evaluate anticanine distemper serum. The complement-fixation titer of antiserum was some indication of protection but a direct relationship could not be established. LAIDLAW and DUNKIN (1931) found that the most effective antiserum was produced in dogs by a massive single dose or closely spaced double doses of formalin-inactivated virus followed by exposure to virulent virus several weeks later and exsanguination 7 to 14 days after the last exposure.

GREEN and CARLSON (1945) reported that CD antiserum of canine origin administered to foxes almost completely neutralized ferret-passaged CDV given 18 days later. OTT et al. (1964) showed that CD antiserum inhibited replication of chicken egg-adapted virus vaccine in dogs when injected up to 20 days later. They also demonstrated that this antiserum, given 2 to 7 days prior to injection of ferrets with 50,000 LD_{50} of ferret-passaged virus, protected a significant number with the greatest protection occurring when antiserum was administered 3 days before challenge virus. These limited studies in ferrets involved a large dose of high titered antiserum against a low dosage of a virulent virus.

BENSON (1960) attempted to correlate neutralizing antibody content in CD antiserum with protection in the dog by challenge with the Snyder Hill virulent strain of CDV. He reported that 6,000 Cornell antibody units per 0.1 ml of serum or antibody concentrate produced in the dog and administered at the rate of 1 ml per lb. (1 ml per 0.45 kg) of body weight were necessary to protect susceptible puppies for 10 days against challenge virus. The Cornell antibody unit was the amount of CD antibody in 0.1 ml of serum expressed as the mean neutralizing dose that will neutralize 300 EID_{50} of Onderstepoort egg-adapted CDV. Although some animals were protected at lower doses, the numbers protected were not sufficient to indicate the use of lower dose levels of serum. Interference in the production of active immunity by egg-modified CDV was encountered when sufficient antibody units had been given 10 days before vaccination.

The procedures of LAIDLAW and DUNKIN (1931) for producing an effective antiserum have not been uniformly adopted by commercial manufacturers because of the cost and the number of susceptible dogs required (PEACOCK, 1966). Producers give large numbers of adult dogs repeated doses of virulent virus, dogs are bled repeatedly, and the serum is pooled. This method of production is still widely used although it does not result in a highly potent antiserum. Unfortunately, it is impossible to increase the antibody titer of most dogs with titers between 1 : 100 and 1 : 1,000 and the percentage with titers above 1 : 1,000 that show a significant rise is extremely low (BAKER et al., 1959). Until the development of the virus-neutralization test, there was no practical way to determine antibody levels in serum. Most commercial antisera do not contain 6,000 Cornell antibody units per 0.1 ml. It is also known that prolonged bleeding will almost invariably result in decreased titers.

PEACOCK (1966) recently reviewed the standard requirements of the United States Department of Agriculture (USDA) for canine distemper antisera produced by U.S. licenses. Alternate antiserum potency tests consisted of the simultaneous serum protection test in animals and its ability to neutralize 100 to 1,000 EID_{50}

of virus at a dilution of not less than 1 : 512. Presently, a standard canine distemper antiserum is furnished by the USDA to manufacturers for neutralization test standardization. This procedure has resulted in an improvement in the titer of marketed antiserum in the U.S. according to PEACOCK. Present standard requirements of the USDA provide a neutralization test in which the ND_{50} dilution of the test serum divided by the ND_{50} of the standard antiserum has the average ratio in two tests of 0.67 or more. Concentrated products are diluted to the equivalent of regular antiserum before twofold serum dilutions are made for the neutralization test. Limited experimental data would suggest that the standard should be increased to have more effective antisera on the market.

The WHO Expert Committee on Biological Standardization recently established the international standard for anti-canine-distemper serum. The Central Veterinary Laboratory, Weybridge, England, arranged a collaborative assay which resulted in the proposed standard (STEWART et al., 1968). Anti-canine-distemper serum was prepared in a horse and tested in vitro in 7 laboratories in 6 countries. The international unit of anti-canine-distemper serum was defined as the activity contained in 0.0897 mg of the international standard of anti-canine-distemper serum. Ampoules containing 1000 international units of freeze-dried serum are available. Dog protection studies with this product were not reported.

F. Epizootiology

The epizootiology of CD was recently reviewed by GORHAM (1966) who has made many notable contributions to this field. Canine distemper has the typical age pattern and incidence for a widespread disease with a long-lasting active immunity. It is enzootic in most areas of the world. Infected animals shed virus in all body excretions (cf., p. 41) and a large variety of animals can be naturally infected by CDV (cf. p. 27). Transmission of virus occurs mostly by aerosol (LAIDLAW and DUNKIN, 1926 a). In spite of very effective attenuated virus vaccines available and extensive vaccination of dogs, CDV is still prevalent and susceptible dogs in dense population areas become infected.

1. Seasonal Prevalence

In his study of the natural history of CD in a large, densely populated area ROCKBORN (1958) used information from practitioners and the Royal Veterinary College in Stockholm about clinical cases of CD. He plotted the monthly mean values of the number of cases and the greatest incidence occurred in the winter. AVON (1963) recorded that most clinical cases were recorded at the onset of inclement weather in the fall. It is rather interesting that seasonal variations were not observed by ERNO and MÖLLER (1961) who used the necropsy records for the period 1950—1957 rather than clinical cases of the Danish Veterinary School. The above studies were conducted with dog populations in temperate climates; unfortunately, there are no reported seasonal prevalence studies for tropical areas. In most countries, there appears to be a constant supply of puppies throughout the course of the year. With a susceptible population always on the scene, it is easy to see why the disease can maintain itself in the dog population. In all likelihood, the attack rate is constant throughout the course of the year but clinical disease manifests itself more frequently during the cold seasons of the year when environmental conditions encourage frank disease. ROCKBORN (1958) estimated that 75 per cent of natural disease in dogs is subclinical in nature.

Table 7. *The Percentage of Distemper-Suscep-tible Dogs in Relation to Their Age*[1]

Age of dog	Per cent susceptible
4—6 months	74
6—12 months	51
1—2 years	37
2—3 years	19
3—4 years	16
4—5 years	6
6—10 years	3—4

[1] HOFFMAN, 1949.

Reprinted with permission from: GORHAM, JOHN R.: Canine Distemper. Advanc. vet. Sci., **6**, 287—351 (1960).

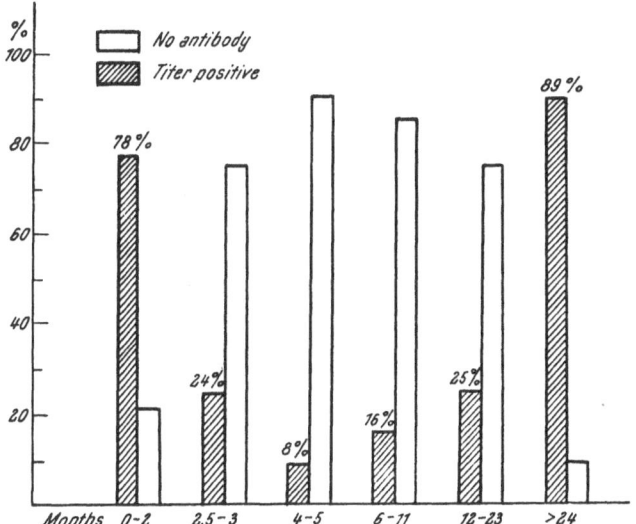

Fig. 30. Distribution of CDV antibody in different age groups of unvaccinated urban dogs (redrawn from ROCK-BORN, 1958 d). Reprinted with permission from: GORHAM, JOHN R.: Advanc. vet. Sci. 6, 287—351 (1960)

2. Age Incidence in Urban Communities

There is general agreement that young dogs are susceptible to CDV when they lose maternal antibody. CARRÉ (1905) and LAIDLAW and DUNKIN (1931) already suggested that temporary protection was afforded young puppies by the milk of immune mothers. HOFFMAN (1949) reported that puppies from immune mothers resisted challenge with virulent virus until they were 6 weeks of age. At 7 weeks, more than half were resistant while at 8 weeks of age, only approximately 30 per cent resisted challenge. He found the highest susceptibility rate in dogs 4—6 months of age with a gradual decline thereafter (Table 7).

A serological study of distemper immunity of an urban unvaccinated dog population was made by ROCKBORN (1958) (Fig. 30). The majority (80 per cent) of the pups newborn to 8 weeks of age had neutralizing antibody. A gradual decline occurred in the 4-to-5 month old group, only 10 per cent had neutralizing antibody. A gradual increase occurred thereafter. Less than 20 per cent of the 6-to-11 month group had antibody and slightly over 20 per cent in the 12-to-23 month group were positive. Eighty-five per cent of the dogs over 24 months had antibody. A CD serological study of a community in the United States was made by CABASSO et al. (1962) and their results were comparable to ROCKBORN's.

GILLESPIE et al. (1956) studied the question of maternal immunity in 95 dogs. All puppies one to 16 weeks of age from susceptible dams were susceptible to CDV. A high percentage of pups died with a hemorrhagic enteritis. Pups from immune dams were more resistant. Nine of 23 five to 8 week old pups showed clinical disease after CDV challenge and only one died, whereas 23 of 25 twelve to 16 week old pups became ill and 16 per cent died.

3. Age Incidence in Isolated Communities

Distemper is enzootic in cities in northern countries such as Greenland and Alaska; however, smaller remote villages do not have a sufficient number of susceptible dogs to maintain the disease, thus, a highly susceptible group of dogs emerges in these villages. The first observation of the dire consequences when CDV invaded dogs of this type was reported by HJORTLUND (1908) describing the disastrous outbreaks in Greenland between 1888 and 1904. Of particular interest is the outbreak in Point Barrow, Alaska, that extended to Anaktuvuk Pass the following year causing the death of 500 dogs (REINHARD, 1953; REINHARD et al., 1955). Dogs of all ages were affected. An outbreak was traced by SOBAUGH (1966, quoted by GORHAM, 1966), from Juneau, Alaska, where the disease is enzootic to the island community of Sitka. Distemper was recognized in unvaccinated dogs in Juneau during the fall, 1965, and first appeared in Sitka in December 1965, where an estimated 500 dogs resided. Between 100 to 200 dogs of all ages died including some 8 and 9 years old. GORHAM (1960) has studied similar outbreaks in dog populations of small, isolated Idaho logging towns and observed similar events as described by REINHARD.

4. The Disease in Wildlife

Little is known about the natural history of the disease in wildlife, but certainly this information would be highly desirable. The wildlife species that are susceptible to CDV were given in an earlier section (cf. p. 27). Few serological studies in wildlife species have been made and more would be useful for increasing our knowledge of the host spectrum. This could also assist in evaluating the transmission of this disease to isolated dog communities by wildlife.

Acknowledgment

The authors would like to acknowledge the contributions of all investigators who supplied information through "personal communication" as recorded, especially R. H. Bussell, J. R. Gorham, A. Koestner, and A. Shishido. Also, the reading and correcting of parts of the manuscript by R. H. Bussell and L. E. Carmichael was greatly appreciated. Many thanks to Miss S. Hanson for typing the manuscript.

References

ACKERMANN, O.: Bessere Immunisierungsmöglichkeiten bei Nerzen gegen Staupe. Dtsch. tierärztl. Wschr. **73**, 11—14 (1966).

ACKERMANN, O.: Early immunization against canine distemper and hepatitis, using combined vaccines. J. Amer. vet. med. Ass. **156**, 1755 (1970).

ACKERMANN, O., und H. SIEBEL: Der Einsatz von Masernvaccinen bei der Schutzimpfung des Hundes. Kleintier-Prax. **13**, 48—53 (1968).

ADAMS, J. M.: Primary virus pneumonitis with cytoplasmic inclusion bodies: Study of epidemic involving thirty-two infants with nine deaths. J. Amer. med. Ass. **116**, 925—933 (1941).

ADAMS, J. M.: Comparative study of canine distemper and a respiratory disease of man. Pediatrics, **11**, 15—27 (1953).

ADAMS, J. M., and D. T. IMAGAWA: Immunological relationship between measles and distemper virus. Proc. Soc. exp. Biol. (N. Y.) **96**, 240—244 (1957).

ADAMS, J. M., D. T. IMAGAWA, S. W. WRIGHT, and G. TARJAN: Measles immunization with live avian distemper virus. Virology **7**, 351—353 (1959).

AKKER, V. D. S.: Hard-pad disease. T. Diergeneesk. **77**, 511—514 (1952).

ALVORD, E. C., W. H. SUDDUTH, S. HRUBY, and K. HUGHES: A search for brain antigens in canine distemper. Neurology **18**, 112 (1968).

ANDERSSON, G.: Studier av antikroppsbildnigen i samband med experitell valpsjuka hos hund. Nord. Vet. Møte. **7**, 129—133 (1954).

ANDREWES, C. H., S. GARD, W. M. HAMMON, F. P. McWHORTER, and V. M. ZHDANOV: Recommendations on virus nomenclature. Virology **21**, 516—517 (1963).

ANGULO, J. J., O. W. RICHARDS, and A. L. ROQUE: Demonstration of viral inclusion bodies in unstained tissue sections with the aid of the phase microscope. I. The inclusion bodies of yellow fever, herpes implex, fowl pox, and distemper. J. Bact. **57**, 297—303 (1949).

Anonym.: Susceptibility of the lesser panda to canine distemper. Internat. Zoo Year Book **2**, 107 (1960). Cited from v. MICKWITZ, Kleintier-Prax. **13**, 80 (1968).

APPEL, M.: Studies on the pathogenesis of canine distemper. Ph. D. Thesis Cornell University (1967).

APPEL, M.: Pathogenesis of canine distemper. Amer. J. vet. Res. **30**, 1167 (1969).

APPEL, M.: Distemper pathogenesis in dogs. J. Amer. vet. med. Ass. **156**, 1681 (1970).

APPEL, M., and O. R. JONES: Use of alveolar macrophages for cultivation of canine distemper virus. Proc. Soc. exp. Biol. (N. Y.) **126**, 571—574 (1967).

APPEL, M., and D. H. PERCY: SV5-like parainfluenza virus in dogs. J. Amer. vet. med. Ass. **156**, 1778 (1970).

APPEL, M., D. H. PERCY, and J. M. GASKIN: Canine distemper virus in domestic cats. (In preparation.)

APPEL, M., P. H. PICKERILL, M. MENEGUS, D. H. PERCY, I. M. PARSONSON, and B. E. SHEFFY. Current status of canine respiratory disease. Gaines Veterinary Symposium (1970).

APPEL, M., B. E. SHEFFY, and D. H. PERCY: Canine distemper virus in domestic pigs. (In preparation.)

ARAKAWA, S., S. MUTO, T. KANEKO, and T. SEKI: Experimental studies on canine distemper (CDV). I. Experiment on the isolation of the virus in mice and embryonated eggs and the relation of the mouse adapted CDV to mouse fixed measles virus and others. Yokohama med. Bull. **10**, 179—189 (1959).

ARMSTRONG, W. H.: Canine distemper in the American badger. Cornell Vet. **32**, 447 (1942).

ARMSTRONG, W. H., and C. G. ANTHONY: An epizootic of canine distemper in a zoological park. Cornell Vet. **32**, 286—288 (1942).

ARMSTRONG, W. H., and T. BURNSTEIN: Neuropathologic changes of experimental distemper in the hamster. Amer. J. vet. Res. **27**, 1083—1091 (1966).

ARNOLD, P., C. BIRNBAUM, H. J. CHRISTOPH, E. G. GRÜNBAUM, M. OETTEL, E. SCHIMKE und I. SOMMER: Klinische Aspekte der Problematik der Staupe *(Febris contagiosa canum)* des Hundes. Mh. Vet.-Med. **23**, 791 (1968).

BAKER, G. A., R. W. LEADER, and J. R. GORHAM: Immune response of ferrets to vaccination with egg-adapted distemper virus. I. Time of development of resistance to virulent distemper virus. Vet. Med. **47**, 463—466 (1952).

BAKER, G. A., J. R. GORHAM, and R. W. LEADER: Studies on an *in ovo* neutralization test for distemper. Amer. J. vet. Res. **15**, 102—107 (1954).

BAKER, J. A.: Heterotypic vaccines: A new concept for prevention of virus diseases in dogs. Proc. 12th Gaines Vet. Symp., Kankakee, Ill. pp. 7—8 (1963).

BAKER, J. A.: Measles vaccine for protection of dogs against canine distemper. J. Amer. vet. med. Ass. **156**, 1743 (1970).

BAKER, J. A., D. S. ROBSON, J. H. GILLESPIE, J. A. BURGHER, and M. R. DOUGHTY: A nomograph that predicts the age to vaccinate puppies against distemper. Cornell Vet., **49**, 158—167 (1959).

BAKER, J. A., B. E. SHEFFY, D. S. ROBSON, and J. GILMARTIN: Response to measles virus by puppies with maternally transferred distemper antibodies. Cornell Vet. **56**, 588—594 (1966).

BALCONI, I. R., J. E. BRAHAM, and R. BRESSANI: Changes in the nitrogen balance and serum proteins during an attack of distemper and coccidiosis in the dog. Cornell Vet. **57**, 429—438 (1967).

BARDACH, M., J. CROS-DECAM et P. GORET: Recherches sur la rougeole. Essais de transmission au chien. C. R. Acad. Sci. (Paris) **225**, 1036—1038 (1947).

BATTELLI, C., e R. SOBRERO: Rapporti immunologici tra il virus della peste bovina e quello del cimurro: Resultati di alcune prove di siero-infezione contro la peste bovina effettuate in Somalia utilizando virus pestoso virulento e siero iperimmune anticimurro. Vet. ital. **12**, 835—843 (1961).

BAUMANN, G.: Zur Diagnose der Staupe mit Hilfe fluoreszierender Antikörper. Mh. Vet.-Med. **22**, 179—185 (1967).

BECH, V.: Relationship between complement-fixing antibodies against measles virus and canine distemper virus. Acta path. microbiol. scand. **50**, 331 (1960).

BELCHER, J.: Certain characteristics of egg-adapted strains of distemper virus. M. S. Thesis, Univ. Wisconsin, 1951.

BENSON, T. F.: The protection of susceptible puppies for ten days against canine distemper using quantitative amounts of antibodies. M. S. Thesis, Cornell University, Ithaca, New York, 1960.

BINDRICH, H.: Beobachtungen bei Staupeviruspassagen an Hunden. Arch. exp. Vet.-Med. **1**, 68—81 (1950 a).

BINDRICH, H.: Untersuchungen über den Virusgehalt des Blutes und der Organe bei Hundestaupe. Arch. exp. Vet.-Med. **2**, 73—78 (1950 b).

BINDRICH, H.: Zur Ausscheidung des Hundestaupevirus mit dem Harn. Arch. exp. Vet.-Med., **3**, 34—38 (1951 a).

BINDRICH, H.: Untersuchungen über die nervöse Staupe des Hundes. Arch. exp. Vet.-Med., **4**, 98—115 (1951 b).

BINDRICH, H.: Untersuchungen über die pH-Resistenz des Virus der Hundestaupe. Arch. exp. Vet.-Med. **4**, 120—126 (1951 c).

BINDRICH, H.: Beitrag zum Wesen der Staupevirusinfektion des Hundes und zu ihrer Bekämpfung. Arch. exp. Vet.-Med. **8**, 131—162, 263—315 (1954).

BINDRICH, H.: Über die Ätiologie der nervösen Erkrankungen des Hundes. Mh. Vet.-Med. **10**, 1—10 (1955).

BINDRICH, H.: Die Virusstaupe des Hundes. Kleintier-Prax. **7**, 161—171, 181—187 (1962).

BINDRICH, H., und H. GRALHEER: Untersuchungen zur Größenbestimmung des Virus der experimentellen Hundestaupe. Arch. exp. Vet.-Med. **8**, 204—211 (1954).

BINDRICH, H., E. KUWERT, H. LINSERT und H. ZIMMERMANN: Zur Staupeerkrankung des Nerzes. Arch. exp. Vet.-Med. **13**, 1—25 (1959).

BINDRICH, H., und D. SCHMIDT: Liquordiagnostik bei experimenteller Staupe des Hundes. Arch. exp. Vet.-Med. **6**, 162—174 (1952).

BINDRICH, H., und D. SCHMIDT: Über die Chloroformresistenz einiger Virusarten (atypische und klassische Geflügelpest, Staupe, Tollwut, Poliomyelitis murium). Arch. exp. Vet.-Med. **9**, 922—934 (1955).

BINN, L. N., G. A. EDDY, E. C. LAZAR, J. HELMS, and T. MURNANE: Viruses recovered from laboratory dogs with respiratory disease. Proc. Soc. exp. Biol. (N. Y.) 126, 140—145 (1967).

BITTLE, J. L.: Newer knowledge on the use of measles vaccine for canine distemper prophylaxis. J. Amer. vet. med. Ass. 156, 1752 (1970).

BITTLE, J. L., C. J. YORK, and J. W. NEWBERNE: Adaptation and modification of a strain of canine distemper virus in tissue culture. Cornell Vet. 51, 359—369 (1961).

BJOTVEDT, G., L. W. GEIB, and P. H. MANN: The role of canine distemper in respiratory disease of non-conditioned laboratory dogs. Lab. Anim. Care 19, 789 (1969).

BLACK, F. L.: Relationship between virus particle size and filterability through Gradocol membranes. Virology 5, 391—392 (1958).

BLACK, F. L., and L. ROSEN: Patterns of measles antibodies in residents of Tahiti and their stability in the absence of re-exposure. J. Immunol. 88, 725 (1962).

BLINZINGER, K., und N. DEUTSCHLÄNDER: Über eigentümliche kristallgitterartige Strukturkomplexe im Gehirn von staupekranken Hunden. Verh. Dtsch. Ges. Path. 53, 283 (1969).

BODIN, S.: Nagra erfarenheter av ympning mot valpsjuka med simultanympämne enlight Laidlaw-Dunkin och ympämne enlight Green. Skand. Vettidskr. 37, 696—715 (1947).

BODINGBAUER, J.: Retention of teeth in dogs as a sequel to distemper infection. Vet. Rec. 72, 636—637 (1960).

BORNSTEIN, M. B., and C. S. RAINE: Experimental allergic encephalitis. Antiserum inhibition of myelination in vitro. Lab. Invest. 23, 536 (1970).

BREAZILE, J. E., B. S. BLAUGH, and N. NAIL: Experimental study of canine distemper myoclonus. Amer. J. vet. Res. 27, 1375—1379 (1966).

BRESNAHAN, M. R., and P. M. NEWBERNE: Interaction of diet and distemper virus infection on lipid metabolism in the dog. Brit. J. exp. Path. 49, 223 (1968).

BROADHURST, J., M. E. MACLEAN, and V. SAURINO: Nasal inclusion bodies in dog distemper. Cornell Vet. 28, 9—15 (1938).

BRUNER, D. W., and J. H. GILLESPIE: Canine distemper. In: Hagan's Infectious Diseases of Domestic Animals. 5th ed., Comstock-Cornell University Press, 1966.

BRYAN, A. H.: Is canine distemper a danger to children? Vet.-Med. 23, 496—497 (1928).

BURGER, D., and J. R. Gorham: Response of ferrets and mink to vaccination with chicken embryo-adapted distemper virus. Arch. ges. Virusforsch. 15, 449 (1964).

BURGHER, J. A., J. A. BAKER, S. SARKAR, V. MARSHALL, and J. H. GILLESPIE: Evaluation of a combined vaccine consisting of modified canine distemper virus and modified infectious canine hepatitis virus for simultaneous immunization of dogs. Cornell Vet. 48, 214—223 (1958).

BURNET, F. M.: Influenza virus infections of the chick embryo lung. Brit. J. exp. Path. 21, 147 (1940).

BUSSEL, R. H.: Canine distemper virus: A review. Tex. Rep. Biol. Med. 24, 386—391 (1966).

BUSSEL, R. H., and D. T. KARZON: Canine distemper virus in chick embryo cell cultures. Plaque assay, growth, and stability. Virology 18, 589—600 (1962).

BUSSEL, R. H., and D. T. KARZON: Canine distemper virus in ferret, dog, and bovine kidney cell cultures. Arch. ges. Virusforsch. 17, 163—182 (1965 a).

BUSSEL, R. H., and D. T. KARZON: Canine distemper virus in primary and continuous cell lines of human and monkey origin. Arch. ges. Virusforsch. 17, 183—202 (1965 b).

BUSSEL, R. H., and D. T. KARZON: Measles — canine distemper — rinderpest group. In: Prier's Basic Medical Virology, pp. 313—336, Williams and Wilkins, Baltimore, 1966.

CABASSO, V. J.: Canine distemper and "hard pad" disease. Proc. Book Amer. vet. med. Ass. 18th Ann. Meet., 150 (1951).

CABASSO, V. J.: Canine distemper and "hard pad" disease. Vet.-Med. 47, 417—423 (1952).

CABASSO, V. J.: The epizootiology of distemper (discussion of). J. Amer. vet. med. Ass. 149, 618—622 (1966).

CABASSO, V. J., J. E. AVAMPATO, K. H. KISER, and M. R. STEBBINS: Further evidence of immunologic dissimilarity of distemper (CD) and measles (M) viruses. Proc. Soc. exp. Biol. (N. Y.) 104, 526—529 (1960).

CABASSO, V. J., R. L. BURCKHARDT, and J. D. LEAMING: The use of an egg-adapted modified canine distemper virus vaccine under experimental conditions and in the field. Vet.-Med. 46, 167—175 (1951).

CABASSO, V. J., and H. R. COX: Propagation of canine distemper virus on the chorio-allantoic membrane of embryonated hen eggs. Proc. Soc. exp. Biol. (N. Y.) 71, 246—250 (1949).

CABASSO, V. J., and H. R. COX: A distemper-like strain of virus derived from a case of canine encephalitis: Its adaptation to the chick embryo and subsequent modification. Cornell Vet. 42, 96—107 (1952).

CABASSO, V. J., J. M. DOUGLAS, M. R. STEBBINS, and H. R. COX: Propagation of canine distemper virus in suckling hamsters. Proc. Soc. exp. Biol. (N. Y.) 88, 199—202 (1955).

CABASSO, V. J., D. W. JOHNSON, M. R. STEBBINS, and H. R. COX: "Atomized" distemper vaccine of avian origin. I. Experimental immunization of ferrets and mink. Amer. J. vet. Res. 18, 414—418 (1957).

CABASSO, V. J., K. KISER, and M. R. STEBBINS: Distemper and measles viruses. I. Lack of immunogenic crossing in dogs and chickens. Proc. Soc. exp. Biol. (N. Y.) 101, 227—230 (1959 a).

CABASSO, V. J., K. KISER, and M. R. STEBBINS: Propagation of canine distemper (CD) virus in tissue culture. Proc. Soc. exp. Biol. (N. Y.) 100, 551—554 (1959 b).

CABASSO, V. J., K. KISER, M. R. STEBBINS, and H. K. COOPER: Canine distemper vaccine of tissue culture origin. Amer. J. vet. Res. 23, 394—402 (1962).

CABASSO, V. J., M. R. STEBBINS, and H. R. COX: Onset of resistance and duration of immunity to distemper in ferrets following a single injection of avianized distemper vaccine. Vet.-Med. 48, 147—150 (1953 a).

CABASSO, V. J., M. R. STEBBINS, and H. R. COX: Active immunization of ferrets by simultaneous injections of avianized canine distemper vaccine and anti-canine distemper hyperimmune serum. Cornell Vet. 43, 179—183 (1953 b).

CABASSO, V. J., M. R. STEBBINS, and H. R. COX: Experimental canine distemper encephalitis and immunization of puppies against it. Cornell Vet. 44, 153—167 (1954).

CAMAND, R., C. MACKOWIAK, L. JOUBERT et P. GORET: Dépistage sérologique comparatif des maladies de Carré et de Rubarth chez le chien. I. Technique de la réaction de fixation du complément. Bull. Acad. vét. Fr. 19, 185—195 (1956).

CAMPBELL, R. S. F.: Encephalitis in canine distemper. Brit. vet. J. 113, 143—162 (1957).

CAMPBELL, R. S. F., W. B. MARTIN, and E. D. GORDON: Toxoplasmosis as a complication of canine distemper. Vet. Rec. 67, 708—713 (1955).

Canine Distemper Symposium. J. Amer. vet. med. Ass. 149, 599—718 (1966).

CAPEN, C. C., and C. R. COLE: Pulmonary lesions in dogs with experimental and naturally occurring toxoplasmosis. Path. Vet. 3, 40 (1966).

CARLSTRÖM, G.: Appearance in children's sera of substances capable of neutralizing canine distemper virus. Acta paediat. (Uppsala) 45, 180—188 (1956).

CARLSTRÖM, G.: Neutralization of canine distemper virus by serum of patients convalescent from measles. Lancet 2, 344 (1957).

CARLSTRÖM, G.: Comparative studies on measles and distemper viruses in suckling mice. Arch. ges. Virusforsch. 8, 527—538 (1958).

CARLSTRÖM, G.: Correlation between canine distemper and measles virus neutralizing capacities in human sera. Arch. ges. Virusforsch. 8, 539—548 (1959).

CARLSTRÖM, G.: Relation of measles to other viruses. Amer. J. Dis. Child. 103, 287 (1962).

CARMICHAEL, L., D. ROBSON, and F. BARNES: Transfer and decline of maternal infectious canine hepatitis antibody in puppies. Proc. Soc. exp. Biol. (N. Y.) 109, 677—681 (1962).

CARRÉ, H.: Sur la maladie des jeunes chiens. C. R. Acad. Sci. (Paris) 140, 689—690, 1489—1491 (1905).

CASCARDO, M. R., and D. T. KARZON: Measles virus giant cell inducing factor (fusion factor). Virology 26, 311—325 (1965).

CELIKER, A., and J. H. GILLESPIE: The effect of temperature, pH, and certain chemicals on egg-cultivated distemper virus. Cornell Vet. 44, 276—280 (1954).

CELLO, R. M., J. E. MOULTON, and S. McFARLAND: The occurrence of inclusion bodies in the circulating neutrophils of dogs with canine distemper. Cornell Vet. 49, 127—146 (1959).

COFFIN, D. L.: Cytopathology of canine distemper studied by the use of fluorescent antibodies. Ann. N. Y. Acad. Sci. 81, 164—171 (1959).

COFFIN, D. L., and C. LIU: Studies on canine distemper infection by means of fluorescein-labeled antibody. II. The pathology and diagnosis of the naturally occurring disease in dogs and the antigenic nature of the inclusion body. Virology 3, 132—145 (1957).

COHRS, P.: Die Entmarkungs-Enzephalitis (hard pad disease) des Hundes. Dtsch. tierärztl. Wschr. 58, 129—134 (1951).

COOPER, P. D.: A chemical basis for the classification of animal viruses. Nature (Lond.) 190, 302—305 (1961).

CORDY, D. R.: Canine encephalomyelitis. Cornell Vet. 32, 11—28 (1942).

CORDY, D. R.: Interstitial pneumonia with giant cells and inclusions. J. Amer. vet. med. Ass. 114, 21—26 (1949).

CORDY, D. R., and J. R. GORHAM: The pathology and etiology of salmon disease in the dog and fox. Amer. J. Path. 26, 617—637 (1950).

CORNWELL, H. J. C., R. S. F. CAMPBELL, J. T. VANTSIS, and W. PENNY: Studies in experimental canine distemper. I. Clinicopathological findings J. comp. Path. 75, 3—17 (1965 a).

CORNWELL, H. J. C., J. T. VANTSIS, R. S. F. CAMPBELL, and W. PENNY: Studies in experimental canine distemper. II. Virology, inclusion body studies and hematology. J. comp. Path. 75, 19—34 (1965 b).

CRANDELL, R. A., W. E. JACKSON, and K. WARMBERG: Serological study for canine distemper and hepatitis in northern Greenland. Nord. Vet.-Med. 18, 162—165 (1966).

CROOK, E.: Pathogenesis and related biological effects of Carré's disease (canine distemper) in certain natural and laboratory hosts. Ph. D. Thesis, Univ. Wisconsin (1957).

CROOK, E., J. R. GORHAM, and S. H. McNUTT: Experimental distemper in mink and ferrets. I. Pathogenesis. Amer. J. vet. Res. 19, 955—957 (1958).

CROOK, E., and S. H. McNUTT: Egg-adaptation of a strain of distemper virus isolated from a raccoon. Amer. J. vet. Res. 19, 223—224 (1958).

CROOK, E., and S. H. McNUTT: Experimental distemper in mink and ferrets. II. Appearance and significance of histopathological changes. Amer. J. vet. Res. 20, 378—383 (1959).

CRUICKSHANK, J. G., A. P. WATERSON, A. D. KANAREK, and D. M. BERRY: The structure of canine distemper virus. Res. Vet. Sci. 3, 485—486 (1962).

CUTCHINS, E. C., and T. R. DAYHUFF: Photoinactivation of measles virus. Virology 17, 420—425 (1962).

CUTLER, R. W. P., and D. R. AVERILL: Cerebrospinal fluid gamma globulins in canine distemper encephalitis. Neurology 19, 1111—1114 (1969).

DALLDORF, G.: The simultaneous occurrence of the viruses of canine distemper and lymphocytic choriomeningitis. A correction of "Canine distemper in the rhesus monkey". J. exp. Med. 70, 19—27 (1939).

DEDIÉ, K.: Die Anwendung der Komplementbindung bei der Hundestaupe. Arch. exp. Vet.-Med. 4, 127—136 (1951).

DEDIÉ, K., J. CHRISTOPH und J. MARTIN: Beitrag zur Staupe bei Silberfüchsen. Arch. exp. Vet.-Med. 11, 689—706 (1957).

DEDIÉ, K., und E. KLAPÖTKE: Die Züchtung des Virus der Hundestaupe im Gewebsexplantat. I. Mitteilung: Die Eignung verschiedener Gewebe. Arch. exp. Vet.-Med. 4, 137—146 (1951).

DEDIÉ, K., und E. KLAPÖTKE: Die Züchtung des Virus der Hundestaupe im Gewebs-explantat. II. Mitteilung: Die Züchtung in laufenden Kulturpassagen. Arch. exp. Vet.-Med. **6**, 57—64 (1952).

DEHAAN, A. B.: Der schlimmste Feind der Nerzzucht-Staupe. Dtsch. Pelztierzüchter **28**, 153 (1954).

DELAY, P. D., S. S. STONE, D. T. KARZON, S. KATZ, and J. ENDERS: Clinical and immune response of alien hosts to inoculation with measles, rinderpest and canine distemper viruses. Amer. J. vet. Res. **26**, 1359—1373 (1965).

DEMONBREUN, W. A.: The histopathology of natural and experimental canine dis-temper. Amer. J. Path. **13**, 187—212 (1937).

DICKSON, M. E., W. M. DICKSON, and J. R. GORHAM: The pH stability of the Wisconsin FXNO strain of egg-adapted distemper virus. Amer. J. vet. Res. **16**, 616—618 (1955).

DONOVAN, C., and R. L. OTT: Distemper inclusion bodies. Vet.-Med. **55**, 53 (1960).

DRÄGER, K., H. FIEGE und R. BARTH: Zur Schutzimpfung gegen Staupe mit lebendem, modifiziertem, eiadaptiertem Staupevirus. Vet. Med. Nachr. **4**, 201—219 (1956).

DRÄGER, K., und R. SCHINDLER: Untersuchungen über den Wert der Komplement-bindungsreaktion (KBR) nach Laidlaw und Dunkin bei der Diagnose der Staupe und bei der Beurteilung des Schutzwertes des Staupeimmunserums. Mh. prakt. Tierheilk. **3**, 262—273 (1951 a).

DRÄGER, K., und R. SCHINDLER: Grundsätzliches zur Handhabung und Auslegung von Staupeexperimenten und einem Modellversuch an Hunden und Frettchen. Mh. prakt. Tierheilk. **3**, 273—282 (1951 b).

DUNKIN, G. W., and P. P. LAIDLAW: Studies in dog distemper. I. Dog distemper in the ferret. J. comp. Path. **39**, 201—212 (1926 a).

DUNKIN, G. W., and P. P. LAIDLAW: Studies in dog distemper. II. Experimental distemper in the dog. J. comp. Path. **39**, 213—221 (1926 b).

ELLIOT, J. A., and W. L. RYAN. Continuous-flow ultracentrifugation of canine distem-per virus and infectious canine hepatitis virus. Appl. Microbiol. **20**, 667 (1970).

ENDERS-RUCKLE, G.: The value of the hemagglutination-inhibition test using the Tween-ether split HA-component of measles virus. Proc. Int. Symp. of Standard of Vaccines against Measles and Serology of Measles and Rubella. Lyon, France, 192—200 (1964).

ERNO, H.: Diagnostizierung der Staupe intra vitam durch Nachweis zytoplasmatischer Einschlußkörperchen im dritten Augenlid. Nord. Vet.-Med. **15**, 21 (1963).

ERNO, H.: On the diagnosis of distemper with special reference to the intraviral demonstration of cytoplasmic inclusion bodies in the third eyelid. Nord. Vet.-Med. **16**, 522 (1964).

ERNO, H., and T. MÖLLER: Epidemiological studies on dog distemper. Nord. Vet.-Med. **13**, 654—674 (1961).

EVANS, J. M., R. GREENWOOD, and S. H. KEEBLE: Protection of dogs against canine distemper. Vet. Rec. **81**, 546—547 (1967).

FAGRAEUS, A., and A. ESPMARK: Use of a mixed haemadsorption method in virus-infected tissue cultures. Nature (Lond.) **190**, 370 (1961).

FAIRCHILD, G. A., M. WYMAN, and E. F. DONOVAN: Fluorescent antibody technique as a diagnostic test for canine distemper infection: Detection of viral antigen in epi-thelial tissues of experimentally infected dogs. Amer. J. vet. Res. **28**, 761—768 (1967).

FAIRCHILD, G. A., S. A. STEINBERG, and D. COHEN: The fluorescent antibody test as a diagnostic test for canine distemper in naturally infected dogs. Cornell Vet. **61**, 214 (1971).

FANKHAUSER, R.: Enzephalitis und hard-pad-Symptom beim Hunde. Schweiz. Arch. Tierheilk. **93**, 715—730, 796—821 (1951).

FARRELL, R. K.: The susceptibility of the American badger to Green's distemperoid vaccine. West. Vet. **4**, 61 (1957).

FARRELL, R. K., J. R. GORHAM, and L. O'NEILL: The response of young mink to varying lengths of exposure to nebulized egg-adapted distemper virus (DV). Vet.-Med. **50**, 412—414 (1955).

FARRELL, R. K., R. L. OTT, and J. R. GORHAM: The failure of egg-propagated distemper virus to interfere with experimental neurotropic distemper in mink. J. Amer. vet. med. Ass. **113**, 269—270 (1958).

FASTIER, L. B.: A complement-fixing antigen from egg-adapted canine distemper virus. Nature (Lond.) **178**, 42—43 (1956).

FENNER, CH., und R. SCHINDLER: Ein Beitrag zur Frage der Hartballenkrankheit (hard pad disease). Mh. prakt. Tierheilk. **4**, 289—300 (1952).

FERRY, N. S.: *Bacillus bronchisepticus (bronchicanis)*; the cause of distemper in dogs and similar disease in other animals. Vet. J. **68**, 376—391 (1912).

FISCHER, K.: Staupe-Enzephalitis bei Dachsen. Schweiz. Arch. Tierheilk. **107**, 87—91 (1965 a).

FISCHER, K.: Einschlußkörperchen bei Hunden mit Staupeenzephalitis und anderen Erkrankungen des Zentralnervensystems. Path. Vet. **2**, 380—410 (1965 b).

FLORIO, R., L. JOUBERT, J. TERRE, J. LAPRAS et G. VAN HAVERBEKE: Epizootiologie comparée de la maladie de Carré et de la rhinoamygdalite du chien dans la région du Sud-Est. Rev. méd. Vét. **116**, 161 (1965).

FONTAINE, M., P. GORET, and A. BRION: Contagious rhinotonsillitis (CRT): A new virus entity unrelated to other infectious diseases in the dog. J. small Anim. Pract. **2**, 71 (1961).

FONTAINE, M., A. RICQ, A. BRION et P. GORET: La rhinoamygdalyte contagieuse du chien. Bull. Acad. vét. Fr. **30**, 315 (1957).

FOX, HERBERT: Diseases in Captive Wild Mammals and Birds. J. B. Lippincott and Co., Philadelphia, Pennsylvania, 1923.

FRASER, G.: The use of rinderpest hyper-immune serums for the detection of canine distemper precipitating antigens. Vet. Rec. **79**, 155 (1966).

FRAUCHIGER, E.: Entmarkungskrankheiten beim Tier. Bull. Schweiz. Akad. med. Wiss. **24**, 66 (1968).

FRAUCHIGER, E., und R. FANKHAUSER: Vergleichende Neuropathologie des Menschen und der Tiere. Springer, Berlin, 1957.

FRAUCHINGER, E., and R. FANKHAUSER: Demyelinating diseases in animals. Handbook of Clinical Neurology, Vol. 13, North-Holland Publ. Co., Amsterdam, 1969.

FUJIE, N., K. KURATA, I. KAIZUKA, and M. SAWADA: Adaptation of avianized distemper virus to suckling mice. Jap. J. vet. Sci. **26**, 273—281 (1964).

GALE, C.: Measles virus for distemper prophylaxis. J. Amer. vet. med. Ass. **156**, 1751 (1970).

GEIGER, W.: Hundestaupe. In: Handbuch der Viruskrankheiten II. Gildemeister, Haagen, Waldmann, Hrsg., 365—379. Fischer, Jena, 1939.

GENTILE, G., M. VENTUROLI, and V. GASPARINI: Paper electrophoresis in canine practice. Vet. ital. **11**, 482 (1960).

GEYER, S., und W. STREHL: Zur Differentialdiagnose der Staupe, Toxoplasmose, Leptospirose und Hepatitis contagiosa canis. Kleintier-Prax. **7**, 133—136 (1962).

GIBSON, J. P.: Distemper virus in brain tissue culture monolayers. Unpublished data. Cited from: STORTS, R. W., A. KOESTNER, R. A. DENNIS, Acta neuropath. (Berl.) **11**, 1 (1968).

GIBSON, J. P., R. A. GRIESEMER, and A. KOESTNER: Experimental distemper in the gnotobiotic dog. J. Path. Vet. **2**, 1—19 (1965).

GILBERT, Y., P. MORNET et Y. GOUEFFON: Comportement humoral du bœuf et du lapin envers l'inoculation du virus de Carré: ses rapports avec l'immunisation contre le virus bovipestique normal ou modifié. Bull. Acad. vét. Fr. **33**, 305 (1960).

GILLESPIE, J. H.: Some preliminary studies on the problem of encephalitis in dogs. Proc. small Anim. Hosp. Ass., 18th Annual Meeting, 164 (1951).

GILLESPIE, J. H.: The virus of canine distemper. In: Comparative Virology. Ann. N. Y. Acad. Sci. **101**, 540—547 (1962).

GILLESPIE, J. H.: A study of inactivated distemper virus in the dog. Cornell Vet. **55**, 3—8 (1965).

GILLESPIE, J. H., J. A. BAKER, J. BURGHER, D. ROBSON, and B. GILMAN: The immune response of dogs to distemper virus. Cornell Vet. **48**, 103—126 (1958).

GILLESPIE, J. H., J. A. BAKER, and G. C. POPPENSIEK: Diarrhea in puppies caused by distemper virus. Ann. N. Y. Acad. Sci. **66**, 204—209 (1956).

GILLESPIE, J. H., A. L. BRUECKNER, J. HEJL, R. JACKSON, R. B. McCLELLAND, and R. L. OTT: Conclusions and recommendations of the panel of the symposium on canine distemper immunization. J. Amer. vet. med. Ass. **149**, 714—717 (1966).

GILLESPIE, J. H., and D. T. KARZON: A study of the relationship between canine distemper and measles in the dog. Proc. Soc. exp. Biol. (N. Y.) **105**, 547—551 (1960).

GILLESPIE, J. H., and C. G. RICKARD: Encephalitis in dogs produced by distemper virus. Amer. J. vet. Res. **17**, 103—108 (1956).

GILLESPIE, J. H., J. I. ROBINSON, and J. A. BAKER: Dual infection of dogs with distemper virus and virus of infectious canine hepatitis. Proc. Soc. exp. Biol. (N. Y.) **81**, 461—463 (1952).

GORET, P., A. BRION et M. FONTAINE: Echec des essais de prévention et de traitment de la maladie de Carré par le sérum contre la peste bovine. Bull. Acad. vét. Fr. **33**, 343—347 (1960).

GORET, P., A. BRION, M. FONTAINE, MME. M. FONTAINE, CH. PILET, M. GIRARD et MME. M. GIRARD: Nouvelles recherches expérimentales sur le virus de la rhino-amygdalite contagieuse du chien. I. Pouvoir pathogène expérimentale. Bull. Acad. vét. Fr. **32**, 625 (1959). II. Pouvoir antigène et immunogène. Bull. Acad. vét. Fr. **32**, 635 (1959).

GORET, P., J. FONTAINE, C. MACKOWIAK, C. PILET et T. CAMARA: Neutralisation du virus de la maladie de Carré par le sérum contre la peste bovine. Bull. Acad. vét. Fr. **32**, 287—296 (1959).

GORET, P., L. A. MARTIN et L. JOUBERT: Essais d'infection et d'immunisation du furet par le virus de Carré adapté au lapin. Bull. Acad. vét. Fr. **25**, 399—404 (1952).

GORET, P., P. MORNET, Y. GILBERT et C. PILET: Immunité croisée entre la maladie de Carré et la peste bovine. C. R. Acad. Sci. (Paris) **245**, 2564—2566 (1957).

GORET, P., P. MORNET, Y. GILBERT et C. PILET: Une curieuse parenté immunologique: Constatation d'une immunité croisée entre la maladie de Carré et la peste bovine (Recherches préliminaires). Bull. Off. Int. Epiz. **49**, 501—506 (1958).

GORET, P., P. MORNET, Y. GILBERT, C. PILET et G. ORTH: Recherches sur l'immunisation croisée «maladie de Carré — peste bovine» chez le lapin. Ann. Inst. Pasteur **98**, 605—610 (1960).

GORET, P., C. PILET, M. GIRARD et T. CAMARA: Apparition et durée de l'immunité contre la maladie de Carré conférée au furet par le virus lapinisé de la peste bovine. Ann. Inst. Pasteur **98**, 610—612 (1960).

GORHAM, J. R.: Pollak's trichrome stain for demonstrating distemper inclusion bodies in tissue sections. Science **107**, 175 (1948).

GORHAM, J. R.: Diseases and parasites of mink. Farmer Bull. No. 2050 USDA (1952).

GORHAM, J. R.: A simple technique for the inoculation of the chorioallantoic membrane of chicken embryos. Amer. J. vet. Res. **18**, 691—692 (1957 a).

GORHAM, J. R.: Egg-propagated distemper virus. Vet.-Med. **52**, 339—346 (1957 b).

GORHAM, J. R.: Canine distemper. In: Advanc. vet. Sci., pp. 287—351. (C. A. BRANDLY and E. L. JUNGHERR, eds.), Academic Press, New York, 1960.

GORHAM, J. R.: The epizootiology of distemper. J. Amer. vet. med. Ass. **149**, 610—622 (1966).

GORHAM, J. R., and C. A. BRANDLY: The transmission of distemper among ferrets and mink. Proc. Book Amer. vet. med. Ass., 90th Ann. Meeting, 129—141 (1953).

GORHAM, J. R., R. K. FARRELL, and R. L. OTT: Preliminary studies on a living virus dust vaccine for distemper. Cornell Vet. **45**, 326—330 (1955).

GORHAM, J. R., R. K. FARRELL, R. L. OTT, and T. PARISOT: Multiplication of attenuated egg-adapted distemper virus in the vaccinated host. Vet.-Med. **52**, 289—292 (1957).

GORHAM, J. R., R. W. LEADER, and J. C. GUTIERREZ: Distemper immunization of ferrets by nebulization with egg-adapted virus. Science **119**, 125—126 (1954 a).

GORHAM, J. R., R. W. LEADER, and J. C. GUITERREZ: Distemper immunization of mink by air-borne infection with egg-adapted virus. J. Amer. vet. med. Ass. **125**, 134—136 (1954 b).

Goss, L. J.: Species susceptibility to the viruses of Carré and feline enteritis. Amer. J. vet. Res. **9**, 65—68 (1948).

Goss, L. W., C. R. Cole, and H. Engel: Inclusion bodies, with special application to clinical diagnosis of canine distemper. J. Amer. vet. med. Ass. **112**, 236—237 (1948).

Gourlay, J. A.: A note on the use of plaque reduction to test serum for canine distemper. Cornell Vet. **60**, 613 (1970).

Green, R. G.: Distemper in the silver fox *(Vulpes vulpes)*. Proc. Soc. exp. Biol. (N. Y.) **23**, 677—678 (1926).

Green, R. G.: Modification of the distemper virus. J. Amer. vet. med. Ass. **95**, 465—466 (1939).

Green, R. G., and W. E. Carlson: The immunization of foxes and dogs to distemper with ferret-passage virus. J. Amer. vet. med. Ass. **107**, 131—142 (1945).

Green, R. G., and C. A. Evans: Rapid diagnosis of canine distemper. Cornell Vet. **29**, 35—40 (1939 a).

Green, R. G., and C. A. Evans: A comparative study of distemper inclusions. Amer. J. Hyg. **29**, 73—87 (1939 b).

Green, R. G., and C. S. Stulberg: Cell-blockade in canine distemper. Proc. Soc. exp. Biol. (N. Y.) **61**, 117—121 (1946).

Green, R. G., and F. S. Swale: Vaccination of dogs with modified distemper virus. J. Amer. vet. med. Ass. **95**, 469—470 (1939).

Greig, A. S.: A pleuro-pneumonia-like organism from dogs. Ph. D. Thesis, Cornell University, Ithaca, N. Y., 1953.

Grünberg, W.: Zur Staupe bei Polarhund und Dingo. Dtsch. tierärztl. Wschr. **66**, 444—447 (1959).

Guarda, F., e U. Dotta: La conferma della diagnosi clinica di cimurro mediante la ricerca dei corpi inclusi nelle cellule epiteliali della congiutiva e della lingua. Ann. Fac. Med. vet. Torino **9**, 323 (1959).

Gutekunst, R. R.: Studies on canine pleuropneumonia-like organism. Ph. D. Thesis, Cornell University, Ithaca, N. Y., 1958.

Gutierrez, J. C., and J. R. Gorham: The adaptation of distemper virus to suckling mice and hamsters. Amer. J. vet. Res. **16**, 325—330 (1955).

Habermann, R. T., C. M. Herman, and F. P. Williams: Distemper in raccoons and foxes suspected of having rabies. J. Amer. vet. med. Ass. **132**, 31—35 (1958).

Hagen, K. W., H. Goto, and J. R. Gorham: Distemper vaccine in pregnant ferrets and mink. Res. Vet. Sci. **11**, 458 (1970).

Haig, D. A.: Preliminary note on the cultivation of Green's distemperoid virus in fertile hen eggs. Onderstepoort J. vet. Sci. Anim. Ind. **23**, 149—155 (1948).

Haig, D. A.: Further observations on the growth of Green's distemperoid virus in developing hen eggs. J. S. Afr. vet. med. Ass. **19**, 73—80 (1949).

Haig, D. A.: Canine distemper-immunization with avianised virus. Onderstepoort J. vet. Res. **27**, 19—53 (1956).

Haig, D. A., B. M. McIntosh, R. B. Cumming, and J. F. D. Hempstead: An outbreak of horsesickness, complicated by distemper, in a pack of fox hounds. J. S. Afr. vet. med. Ass. **27**, 245—249 (1956).

Hammerton, A. C.: Proc. zoological Society of London **2**, 443 (1937). Cited after Armstrong and Anthony, 1942.

Hara, T.: Studies on canine distemper. I. Sensibility of adult hamsters. NIBS (Nippon Inst. Biol. Sci.) Bull. biol. Res. **2**, 58—66 (1957).

Hardenbergh, J. G.: The significance of *Bacillus bronchisepticus* in cases of canine distemper. J. Amer. vet. med. Ass. **68**, 309—320 (1925).

Harrison, M. J.: Canine distemper virus cultured in a diploid monkey cell strain. Nature (Lond.) **201**, 1055 (1964).

Harrison, M. J., D. T. Oxer, and F. A. Smith: The virus of canine distemper in cell culture. II. Effect of serial passage in ferret kidney cell cultures and BS-C-1 cultures on the virulence of canine distemper virus. J. comp. Path. **78**, 133—139 (1968 b).

HARRISON, M. J., F. A. SMITH, and J. J. GRAYDON: The virus of canine distemper in cell culture. I. Adaptation of canine distemper virus to growth and serial passage in ferret kidney cell cultures and in BS-C-1 cell cultures. J. comp. Path. **78**, 121—131 (1968 a).

HEMBOLDT, C. F., and E. L. JUNGHERR: Distemper complex in wild carnivores simulating rabies. Amer. J. vet. Res. **16**, 463—469 (1955).

HOEKENGA, M. T., A. J. F. SCHWARZ, H. C. PALMA, and P. A. BOYER: Experimental vaccination against measles. II. Tests of live measles and live distemper vaccine in human volunteers during a measles epidemic in Panama. J. Amer. med. Ass. **173**, 868 (1960).

HOFFMAN, F.: Studies on distemper. Acta vet. hung. **1**, 89—92 (1949).

HOLMES, F. O.: Order Virales. The filterable viruses (Supplement II). In: Bergey's Manual of Determinative Bacteriology (R. D. BREED, E. G. D. MURRAY, and A. P. HITCHENS, eds.), 6th ed., pp. 1127—1286. Williams & Wilkins, Baltimore, Maryland, 1948.

HOPPER, P. K.: The preparation of canine distemper virus in tissue culture. J. comp. Path. **69**, 78—86 (1959 a).

HOPPER, P. K.: Investigations on neutralizing antibody to canine distemper virus in human serum from different countries. Acta paediat. (Uppsala) **48**, 43—49 (1959 b).

HORSFALL, F. L., and E. H. LENNETTE: The synergism of human influenza and canine distemper viruses in ferrets. J. exp. Med. **72**, 247—259 (1940).

HORTA-BARBOSA, L., D. A. FUCCILLO, W. T. LONDON, J. T. JABBOUR, W. ZEMAN, and J. L. SEVER: Isolation of measles virus from brain cell cultures of two patients with subacute sclerosing panencephalitis. Proc. exp. Biol. (N. Y.) **132**, 272—277 (1969).

HSIUNG, G., and H. J. STAFSETH: Canine distemper. I. Bacteriological studies. Cornell Vet. **42**, 223—231 (1952).

HUMMON, O. J., and F. R. BUSHNELL: Tissue vaccine in the control of mink distemper. J. Amer. vet. med. Ass. **102**, 102—105 (1943).

HUNT, R. D., J. F. FERRELL, S. W. THOMPSON, and G. WALTON: A histochemical comparison of the inclusion bodies of canine distemper and infectious canine hepatitis. Amer. J. vet. Res. **24**, 1248—1255 (1963).

HURST, E. W., B. T. COOKE, and P. MELVIN: "Nervous distemper" in dogs. A pathological and experimental study, with some reference to demyelinating diseases in general. Aust. J. exp. Biol. med. Sci. **21**, 115—126 (1943).

IMAGAWA, D. T.: Comparative studies of measles, distemper and rinderpest viruses. Bact. Proc. 105 (1965 a).

IMAGAWA, D. T.: Propagation of rinderpest virus in suckling mice and its comparison to murine adapted strains of measles and distemper. Arch. ges. Virusforsch. **17**, 203—215 (1965 b).

IMAGAWA, D. T.: Relationships among measles, canine distemper, and rinderpest viruses. Progr. med. Virol. **10**, 160—193 (1968).

IMAGAWA, D. T., and J. M. ADAMS: Propagation of measles virus in suckling mice. Proc. Soc. exp. Biol. (N. Y.) **98**, 567—569 (1958).

IMAGAWA, D. T., C. D. BAIRD, and J. M. ADAMS: Measles and distemper viruses in continuously cultured dog kidney cells. Fed. Proc. **22**, 488 (1963).

IMAGAWA, D. T., P. GORET, and J. M. ADAMS: Immunological relationship of measles, distemper, and rinderpest viruses. Proc. nat. Acad. Sci. (Wash.) **46**, 1119—1123 (1960).

IMAGAWA, D. T., M. YOSHIMORI, S. W. WRIGHT, and J. M. ADAMS: Serum neutralization of distemper virus in chick embryos. Proc. Soc. exp. Biol. (N. Y.) **87**, 2—5 (1954).

INNES, J. R. M.: Demyelinating diseases of animals. II. The relation of distemper infection to the etiology of canine encephalopathies. Vet.-Med. **44**, 421 and 467 (1949).

INNES, J. R. M.: The relation of distemper infection to the aetiology of canine encephalopathies. Vet. Rec. **61**, 73 (1949).

INNES, J. R. M., and L. Z. SAUNDERS: Diseases of the central nervous system of domesticated animals and comparisons with human neuropathology. Advanc. vet. Sci. **3**, 33—196 (1957).

INNES, J. R. M., and L. Z. SAUNDERS: Comparative Neuropathology. Academic Press, New York, 1962.

ISHI, S., G. TOKIDA, and M. WATANABE: Analysis of rinderpest virus antigen. I. Results of the diffusion precipitation test in agar gel. Nat. Inst. Anim. Hlth Quart. **4**, 205—213 (1964).

JACOBY, R. O., and R. A. GRIESEMER: Effect of adrenalectomy on the lymphoid lesions in dogs with experimentally induced canine distemper. Amer. J. vet. Res. **31**, 1825 (1970).

JENNER, E. (1809) (cited by H. KIRK): Canine Distemper, its Complications, Sequelae and Treatment. 1st ed., Baillère, Tindall and Cox, London, 1922.

JOHNSON, D. W., V. J. CABASSO, K. HUFFMAN, and M. R. STEBBINS: "Atomized" distemper vaccine of avian origin. II. Field experience in mink. Amer. J. vet. Res. **18**, 668—671 (1957).

JOHNSON, R. V., C. J. YORK, V. B. ROBINSON, A. H. BRUECKNER, and G. R. BURCH: Immunology of canine distemper. Vet. Med. **54**, 405—412 (1959).

JUBB, K.V.F., and P. C. KENNEDY: Pathology of Domestic Animals. Academic Press 1963.

JUBB, K. V., L. Z. SAUNDERS, and H. V. COATES: The intraocular lesions of canine distemper. J. comp. Path. **67**, 21—29 (1957).

KANTOROWICZ, R.: Experimentelle Untersuchungen über die Hundestaupe und deren Vorbeugung durch eine neue Schutzimpfung. Arch. Tierheilk. **66**, 203 (1933). Cited by BINDRICH, H.: Arch. exp. Vet.-Med. **8**, 263 (1954).

KARSTADT, L., and J. BUDD: Distemper in raccoons characterized by giant cell pneumonitis. Canad. vet. J. **5**, 326—330 (1964).

KARZON, D. T.: Studies on a neutralizing antibody against canine distemper virus found in man. Pediatrics **16**, 809—818 (1955).

KARZON, D. T.: Measles virus. Ann. N. Y. Acad. Sci. **101**, 527—539 (1962).

KARZON, D. T., and R. H. BUSSELL: Cytopathic effect of canine distemper virus in tissue culture. Science **130**, 1708—1709 (1959).

KARZON, D. T., J. H. GILLESPIE, and R. H. BUSSELL: Use of cell culture adapted canine distemper virus in the complement-fixation test. Amer. J. vet. Res. **22**, 1069—1073 (1961).

KASZA, L.: Recovery of canine distemper virus from subcultured primary dog kidney cell culture. Res. vet. Sci. **9**, 187—188 (1968).

KASZA, L., and R. A. GRIESEMER: The production of cytopathic changes in canine cell lines by infectious agents. Path. Vet. **4**, 378—390 (1967).

KEEBLE, S. A.: Living vaccines for the prevention of respiratory virus diseases. Proc. roy. Soc. Med. **55**, 847 (1962).

KEEP, J. M., J. F. STEEL, and J. H. WHITTEM: A clinical, pathological and experimental study of a meningitic syndrome in dogs. Aust. vet. J. **26**, 330—337 (1950).

KEYMER, I. F., and H. B. G. EPPS: Canine distemper in the family Mustelidae. Vet. Rec. **85**, 204 (1969).

KILHAM, L.: Serological studies of canine distemper-complement fixation with spleen antigens. Amer. J. vet. Res. **17**, 398—401 (1956).

KILHAM, L., R. T. HABERMAN, and C. M. HERMAN: Jaundice and bilirubinemia as manifestations of canine distemper in raccoons and ferrets. Amer. J. vet. Res. **17**, 144—148 (1956).

KILHAM, L., and C. M. HERMAN: Isolation of an agent causing bilirubinemia and jaundice in raccoons. Proc. Soc. exp. Biol. (N. Y.) **85**, 272—275 (1954).

KIMES, R. C., and R. N. BUSSELL: The nucleic acid type and effect of pH and hydroxylamine of canine distemper virus. Arch. ges. Virusforsch. **24**, 387—395 (1968).

KIRK, H.: Canine Distemper, its Complications, Sequelae and Treatment. 1st ed., Baillère, Tindall and Cox, London, 1922.

KLAPÖTKE, E.: Versuche zur Vermehrung des Staupevirus im Mäusegehirn. Arch. exp. Vet.-Med. **7**, 85—93 (1953).

KOESTNER, A., and J. F. LONG: Ultrastructure of canine distemper virus in explant tissue cultures of canine cerebellum. Lab. Invest. **23**, 196 (1970).

KOPROWSKI, H.: Counterparts of human viral disease in animals. Ann. N. Y. Acad. Sci. **70**, 369—381 (1958).

KOPROWSKI, H., G. A. JERVIS, T. R. JAMES, R. L. BURKHART, and G. C. POPPENSIEK: A study of canine encephalitis. Amer. J. Hyg. **51**, 63—75 (1950).

KRETSCHMAR, CH.: Zur pathologischen Histologie des Zentralnervensystems bei der nervösen Staupe. Zbl. Vet.-Med. **1**, 366—382 (1954).

KRETSCHMAR, CH.: Zur Frage der Einschlußkörperchen bei der Staupe des Nerzes. Mh. Tierheilk. **7**, 173—180 (1955).

KURATA, K., I. KAIZUKA, and N. FUJIE: Studies on the complement fixation test of distemper virus. I. Use of suckling mouse brain as antigen. Jap. Ann. Rep. Nat. Vet. Assay Lab. **3**, 37—49 (1963).

LAIDLAW, P. P.: Dog distemper. In: "A System of Bacteriology", Vol. 7. Medical Research Council, London 232—243 (1930).

LAIDLAW, P. P., and G. W. DUNKIN: Studies in dog distemper. II. Experimental distemper in the dog. J. comp. Path. **39**, 3, 213—221 (1926 a).

LAIDLAW, P. P., and G. W. DUNKIN: Studies in dog distemper. III. The nature of the virus. J. comp. Path. **39**, 222—230 (1926 b).

LAIDLAW, P. P. and G. W. DUNKIN: A report upon the cause and prevention of dog distemper. Brit. vet. J. **84**, 596—637 (1928 a).

LAIDLAW, P. P., and G. W. DUNKIN: Studies in dog distemper. IV. The immunization of ferrets against dog distemper. J. comp. Path. **41**, 1—17 (1928 b).

LAIDLAW, P. P., and G. W. DUNKIN: Studies in dog distemper. V. The immunization of dogs. J. comp. Path. **41**, 209—227 (1928 c).

LAIDLAW, P. P., and G. W. DUNKIN: Studies in dog distemper. VI. Dog distemper antiserum. J. comp. Path. **44**, 1—25 (1931).

LARIN, N. M.: Canine distemper virus complex. Nature (Lond.) **173**, 174—176 (1954).

LARIN, N. M.: Canine distemper virus in the ferret. J. comp. Path. **65**, 325—333 (1955).

LARIN, N. M., and S. F. J. HODGMAN: Modern approach to canine distemper virus and its practical application. Vet. Rec. **66**, 339—348 (1954).

LARIN, N. M., and W. R. WOOLDRIDGE: A critical approach to canine virus distemper. Brit. vet. J. **113**, 191—202 (1957).

LASFÁRGUES, E.: Essais de culture du virus de la maladie de Carré sur membranes chorio-allantoides et sur tissues embryonnaires de poulet. Ann. Inst. Pasteur **84**, 703—710 (1953).

LAUDER, I. M., W. B. MARTIN, E. D. GORDON, D. D. LAWSON, R. S. F. CAMPBELL, and A. M. WATRACH: A survey of canine distemper. Vet. Rec. **66**, 607—611, 623—631 (1954).

LAWN, A. M.: Ultrastructural features of canine distemper virus infection of the chorioallantoic membrane of the hen's egg. J. gen. Virol. **8**, 157 (1970).

LENTZ, O.: Über spezifische Veränderungen an den Ganglienzellen wut- und staupe-kranker Tiere. Z. Hyg. Infekt.-Kr. **62**, 63 (1909).

LEWIS, G.: An outbreak of infectious canine hepatitis complicated with distemper. N. Amer. Vet. **31**, 743—744 (1950).

LIGNIÈRES, J.: Sur la maladie des chiens et le virus filtrant de Carré. Bull. Soc. méd. vét. **60**, 622—630 (1906).

LINDGREN, A. N. O.: Studier över cytoplasmatiska inklusioner vid valpsjuka hos hund. Nord. Vet.-Med. **3**, 403—422 (1951).

LIU, C.: Relationship of viral antigens to inclusion bodies. Ann. N. Y. Acad. Sci. **81**, 193—196 (1959).

LIU, C., and D. L. COFFIN: Studies on canine distemper infection by means of fluorescein-labeled antibody. I. The pathogenesis, pathology, and diagnosis of the disease in experimentally infected ferrets. Virology **3**, 115—131 (1957).

LO, J. P., W. M. DICKSON, and J. R. GORHAM: Errors in distemper virus titrations performed in embryonated eggs. Arch. ges. Virusforsch. **15**, 74—90 (1965).

Lo, J. P., Ş. E. Svehag, and J. R. Gorham: Thermostability of distemper virus and its neutralization by antibody. Acta vet. scand. **6**, 329 (1965 a).

Lo, J. P., S. E. Svehag, and J. R. Gorham: Sensitivity and error limits of two tests for distemper virus neutralizing antibody: A conventional neutralization test and the "single dilution-probit test". Acta vet. scand. **6**, 341—352 (1965 b).

Lobaugh, C. (cited by J. R. Gorham): The epizootiology of distemper. J. Amer. vet. med. Ass. **149**, 610—618 (1966).

Lockhart, A., J. D. Ray, and J. S. Barbee: Immunity against canine distemper. A report of the development of a new immunizing agent of high efficiency. J. Amer. vet. med. Ass. **67**, 668—670 (1925).

Lou, T. Y., and H. A. Wenner: Natural and experimental infection of the dog with reovirus type 1: Pathogenicity of the strain for other animals. Amer. J. Hyg. **77**, 293—304 (1963).

Lucam, F., et P. Goret: Ovoculture du virus de la maladie de Carré. C. R. Acad. Sci. (Paris) **233**, 107—109 (1951).

Lührs: Hundestaupe. Z. Vetk. **38**, 129 (1926). Cited from H. Bindrich: Arch. exp. Vet.-Med. **8**, 263 (1954).

Lwoff, A., R. Horne, and R. Tournier: A system of viruses. Cold Spr. Harb. Symp. quant. Biol. **27**, 51—55 (1962).

MacIntyre, A. B., D. J. Trevan, and R. Montgomerie: Observations on canine encephalitis. Vet. Rec. **60**, 635—642 (1948).

Maestrone, G.: Demonstration of leptospiral and viral antigens in formalin-fixed tissues. Nature (Lond.) **197**, 409—410 (1963).

Mansey, W.: General discussion to McIntyre, A. B., D. J. Trevan, and R. F. Montgomerie (1948). Vet. Rec. **60**, 642—643 (1948).

Mansi, W.: The isolation of a neurotropic virus from a dog suffering from the socalled nervous distemper. Brit. vet. J. **107**, 214—229 (1951).

Mansi, W.: The canine distemper complex. State vet. J. **7**, 22—26 (1952).

Mansi, W.: The value of the complement-fixation test in the study of canine distemper complex and Rubarth's disease. J. comp. Path. **65**, 291—308 (1955).

Mansi, W.: The study of some viruses by the plate gel diffusion precipitin test. J. comp. Path. **67**, 297—303 (1957).

Mansi, W.: Slide gel diffusion precipitin test. Nature (Lond.) **181**, 1289—1290 (1958).

Mantovani, A.: Coltura del virus del cimurro del cane in embrione di pollo. Vet. ital. **5**, 19—29 (1954 a).

Mantovani, A.: Sulla prova di neutralizzazione del virus di Carré in embrione di pollo. Riv. med. vet. zootecn. **6**, 289—302 (1954 b).

Marjanovic, D.: Veränderungen der Transaminaseaktivität im Liquor cerebrospinalis und im Blutserum von an Staupe erkrankten Hunden. Arch. exp. Vet.-Med. **23**, 253 (1969).

Markiewicz, K.: Examination of the blood and cerebrospinal fluid of dogs with the nervous form of distemper. Med. weteryn. **21**, 528—532 (1965).

Martin, L. A.: Maladie de Carré à forme nerveuse. Transmission du virus au lapin. Bull. Acad. vét. Fr. **23**, 291 (1950).

Martin, L. A.: La sensibilité du singe marocain *Macaca sylvanus* (Linné, 1758) au virus de Carré. Bull. Acad. vét. Fr. **23**, 457 (1950).

Martin, L. A.: Sensibilité du furet au virus de Carré administré par aerosols. Bull. Acad. vét. Fr. **24**, 339—340 (1951).

Martinaglia, G.: S. Afr. J. Sci. **33** (1937). Cited after Armstrong and Anthony (1942).

Matthias, D.: Zur Anwendung der Immunhistologie in der Veterinär-Pathologie. Dtsch. tierärztl. Wschr. **73**, 430 (1966).

McGovern, V. J., J. D. Steel, B. D. Wyke, and M. E. Dodson: Canine encephalitis causing a syndrome characterised by tremor. Aust. J. exp. Biol. med. Sci. **28**, 433—447 (1950).

McGowan, J. P.: Some observations on a laboratory epidemic, principally among dogs and cats in which the animals affected presented the symptoms of the disease called "distemper". J. Path. Bact. **15**, 372—426 (1911).

McGrath, J. T.: Distemper complex. In: "Neurologic Examination of the Dog," 2nd ed., pp. 127—136, Lea & Febiger, Philadelphia, Pennsylvania, 1960.

McManus, K. P.: Experiences with measles virus in canine distemper prophylaxis. Aust. vet. J. **44**, 231 (1968).

Mebus, C. A., and E. M. Coles: Serum glycoprotein alterations in experimental encephalitic canine distemper. Cornell Vet. **55**, 453—461, 462—471 (1965).

Mebus, C. A., and E. M. Coles: Measles-canine distemper relationships. The effect of measles virus and their influence on subsequent challenge with Snyder Hill distemper virus. Cornell Vet. **56**, 85—103 (1966).

Melnick, J. L., and R. M. McCombs: Classification and nomenclature of animal viruses. Progr. med. Virol. **8**, 400—409 (1966).

Mickwitz, C. U. v.: Zur Staupe der Kleinbären (procyoniden). Kleintier-Prax. **13**, 80—90 (1968).

Mickwitz, C. U. v., und H. D. Schröder: Staupeinfektion beim Katzenbär *(Ailurus fulgens)*. Verh.-Ber. IX. Internationales Symposium über Erkrankungen der Zootiere, Prag 1967, pp. 215—217. Akad. Verlag Berlin, 1967. Cited from v. Mickwitz, 1968.

Mickwitz, C. U. v., und H. D. Schröder: Histologische, fluoreszenzserologische und histochemische Untersuchungen zum Verhalten der Einschlußkörperchen bei der Staupe des Hundes. Zbl. Vet.-Med. B. **15**, 453 (1968).

Middlebrook, G.: An apparatus for airborne infection of mice. Proc. Soc. exp. Biol. (N. Y.) **80**, 105—110 (1952).

Millian, S., J. Maisel, C. H. Kempe, S. Plotkin, J. Pagano, and J. Warren: Antibody response of man to canine distemper virus. J. Bact. **79**, 616—618 (1960).

Mitscherlich, E.: Über Züchtungsversuche des Virus der Hundestaupe. Dtsch. tierärztl. Wschr. **46**, 497—502 (1938).

Möller, T.: On the pathogenesis of central nervous system changes in canine toxoplasmosis. Acta neuropath. (Berl.), Suppl. 1, 26—32 (1962).

Möller, T., and S. W. Nielsen: Toxoplasmosis in distemper susceptible carnivora. Path. Vet. **1**, 189—203 (1964).

Momberg-Jørgensen, H. C.: Hvalpesygestudier I. Infections-og vakcinations-forsog pa mink. Nord. Vet.-Med. **1**, 377—387 (1949).

Momberg-Jørgensen, H. C.: Toxoplasmose i forbindelse med hvalpesyge hos minken. Nord. Vet.-Med. **8**, 239—242 (1956).

Mornet, P., P. Goret et Y. Gilbert: Immunité croisée entre la maladie de Carré et la peste bovine. Bull. Epiz. Dis. Afr. **7**, 255—263 (1959 a).

Mornet, P., P. Goret, Y. Gilbert et Y. Goueffon: Nouvelles recherches sur l'immunisation contre la peste bovine à l'aide du virus de la maladie de Carré. C. R. Acad. Sci. (Paris) **248**, 2815—2817 (1959 b).

Mornet, P., P. Goret, Y. Gilbert et Y. Goueffon: Sur les relations croisées des charactères antigènes et immunogènes des virus de la maladie de Carré, et de la peste bovine. État actuel de recherches. Rev. Élev. **13**, 5—25 (1960).

Morris, J. A., C. G. Aulisio, and J. M. McCown: A complement-fixation test for canine distemper. Cornell Vet. **45**, 182—189 (1955).

Morris, J. A., D. R. Coburn, and J. R. O'Connor: Rapid protection of ferrets against fully virulent distemper virus with nebulized attenuated distemper virus. Cornell Vet. **44**, 198—207 (1954).

Morse, H. G., T. L. Chow, and C. A. Brandly: Propagation of a strain of egg-adapted distemper virus in suckling mice. Proc. Soc. exp. Biol (N. Y.) **84**, 10—12 (1953).

Motohashi, T., H. Nakagawa, and T. Okada: Fluorescent antibody technique in diagnosis of canine distemper. Vet. Med. **64**, 1057 (1969).

Motohashi, T., K. Shigeru, and J. Nakamura: Adaptation of a strain of egg-adapted canine distemper virus to weanling and adult hamsters. Amer. J. vet. Res. **25**, 825 (1964).

Motohashi, T., and M. Tajima: Isolation of a herpes virus from a diseased adult dog in Japan. Jap. J. vet. Sci. **28**, 307—314 (1966).

MOULTON, J. E.: Fluorescent antibody studies of demyelination in canine distemper Proc. Soc. exp. Biol. (N. Y.) **91**, 460—464 (1956).

MOULTON, J. E., and C. H. BROWN: Antigenicity of canine distemper inclusion bodies as demonstrated by fluorescent antibody technic. Proc. Soc. exp. Biol. (N. Y.) **86**, 99—102 (1954).

MOURA, R. A., and J. WARREN: Subclinical infection of dogs by canine-adapted measles virus evidenced by their subsequent immunity to canine distemper virus. J. Bact. **82**, 702—705 (1961).

MÜLLER, R. M.: Modern veterinary practice reference and data service H-2-64 (1962). Cited by v. MICKWITZ (1968).

NEMO, G. T., and E. C. CUTCHINS: Photoinactivation of canine distemper virus (CDV). Fed. Proc. **24**, 319 (1965).

NEMO, G. T., and E. C. CUTCHINS: Effect of visible light on canine distemper virus. J. Bact. **91**, 798—802 (1966).

NEWBERNE, P. M.: Overnutrition on resistance of dogs to distemper virus. Fed. Proc. **25**, 1701 (1966).

NICOLLE, C.: La maladie du jeune âge des chiens est transmissible expérimentalement a l'homme sous forme inapparente. Arch. Inst. Pasteur Tunis, **20**, 321—323 (1931).

NORRBY, E.: Measles. In: Recent Advances in Medical Microbiology (A. P. WATERSON, ed.), J. & A. Churchill, Ltd., 1967.

NORRBY, E., B. FRIDING, G. ROCKBORN, and S. GARD: The ultrastructure of canine distemper virus. Arch. ges. Virusforsch. **13**, 335—344 (1963).

OTT R. L.: Comments on heterotypie (measles) vaccine. J. Amer. vet. med. Ass. **149**, 692 (1966).

OTT, R. L., and J. R. GORHAM: The response of newborn and young ferrets to intra-nasal administration with egg-adapted distemper virus. Amer. J. vet. Res. **16**, 571—572 (1955).

OTT, R. L., J. R. GORHAM, and R. K. FARRELL: The effect of dilution of egg-adapted distemper virus on the immune response in ferrets and dogs. N. Amer. Vet. **38**, 219—222 (1957).

OTT, R. L., J. R. GORHAM, and R. K. FARRELL: Note on the use of antiserum and live distemper virus vaccination. Aust. vet. J. **40**, 267—268 (1964).

OTT, R. L., J. R. GORHAM, and J. C. GUTIERREZ: Distemper in dogs. I. Virus neutra-lizing antibodies in serum collected from healthy dogs. J. Amer. vet. med. Ass. **126**, 290—293 (1955).

OTT, R. L., J. R. GORHAM, and J. C. GUTIERREZ: Distemper in dogs. II. The response to vaccination. Amer. J. vet. Res. **18**, 375—381 (1957).

OTT, R. L., S. E. SVEHAG, and D. BURGER: Resistance to experimental distemper in ferrets following the use of killed tissue vaccine. West. Vet. **6**, 107—111 (1959).

PAGE, W. G., and R. G. GREEN: An improved diagnostic stain for distemper inclusions. Cornell Vet. **32**, 265—268 (1942).

PALM, C. R., and F. L. BLACK: A comparison of canine distemper among ferrets and mink. Proc. Book AVMA 90th Ann. Meet. 129—141 (1961 a).

PALM, C. R., and F. L. BLACK: A comparison of canine distemper and measles viruses. Proc. Soc. exp. Biol. (N. Y.) **107**, 588—590 (1961 b).

PARKER, R. L., V. J. CABASSO, D. J. DEAN, and E. L. CHEATUM: Serologic evidence of certain virus infections in wild animals. J. Amer. vet. med. Ass. **138**, 437—440 (1961).

PATERSON, P. Y.: Experimental allergic encephalomyelitis and autoimmune disease. Advanc. Immunol. **5**, 131 (1966).

PAYNE, L. N., P. M. BIGGS, and R. C. CHUBB: Contamination of egg adapted canine distemper vaccine by avian leukosis virus. Vet. Rec. **78**, 45 (1966).

PEACOCK, G. V.: Heterotypic virus vaccines. J. Amer. vet. med. Ass. **149**, 675 (1966).

PECKHAM, J. C.: Pathogenesis of the lesions of the central nervous system in canine distemper. Ph. D. Thesis, Washington State University, 1967.

PETERS, J., und S. YAMAGIWA: Zur Histopathologie der Staupeenzephalitis der Hunde und der epizootischen Enzephalitis der Silberfüchse. Arch. wiss. prakt. Tierheilk. **70**, 138—152 (1936).

PHILLIPS, L. A., and R. H. BUSSELL: Biochemical and biophysical properties of canine distemper virus. I. Nucleic acid studies. Submitted for publication (1971 a).

PHILLIPS, L. A., and R. H. BUSSELL: Biochemical and biophysical properties of canine distemper virus. II. Buoyant density studies. Submitted for publication (1971 b).

PIAT, B. L.: Susceptibility of young lions to dog distemper. Bull. Serv. Elev. Indust. Anim. A. O. F. 3 (1950). Discussion to J. R. GORHAM, 1966.

PIERCY, S. E.: An appraisal of the value and method of use of living attenuated canine distemper vaccines. Vet. Rec. 73, 944—999 (1961).

PIERCY, S. E.: Resistance of egg-adapted canine distemper virus to formalin. Vet. Rec. 74, 590 (1962).

PIERCY, S. E., and R. F. SELLERS: Antibody response to a combined living attenuated distemper-hepatitis vaccine. Res. vet. Sci. 1, 84 (1960).

PINKERTON, H.: Immunological and histological studies on mink distemper. J. Amer. vet. med. Ass. 96, 347—355 (1940).

PINKERTON, H., W. L. SMILEY, and W. A. D. ANDERSON: Giant cell pneumonia with inclusions. A lesion common to Hecht's disease, distemper and measles. Amer. J. Path. 21, 1—23 (1945).

PLOWRIGHT, W.: Rinderpest virus. Ann. N. Y. Acad. Sci. 101, 548—563 (1962).

PLOWRIGHT, W.: Rinderpest Virus. Virology Monographs No. 3, Springer-Verlag, Wien-New York, 1968.

PLOWRIGHT, W., J. G. CRUIKSHANK, and A. P. WATERSON: The morphology of rinderpest virus. Virology 17, 118—122 (1962).

PLUMMER, P. J. G.: Preliminary studies of distemper virus on the chorio-allantoic membrane of the developing egg. Canad. J. comp. Med. vet. Sci. 3, 96—100 (1939).

POLDING, J. B., and R. M. SIMPSON: A possible immunological relationship between canine distemper and rinderpest. Vet. Rec. 69, 582—584 (1957).

POLDING, J. B., R. M. SIMPSON, and G. R. SCOTT: Links between canine distemper and rinderpest. Vet. Rec. 71, 643—645 (1959).

POLSON, A., and W. D. MALHERBE: Changes in the electrophoretic pattern of serum of dogs suffering from various diseases. Onderstepoort J. vet. Res. 25, 13 (1952).

POSTE, G.: Increased growth of viruses in lymphocytes treated with heterologous antilymphocyte serum. Transplantation 10, 106 (1970).

POSTE, G.: The growth and cytopathogenicity of virulent and attenuated strains of canine distemper virus in dog and ferret macrophages. J. comp. Path. 81, 49 (1971).

POTEL, K.: Histopathologie der Hundestaupe mit besonderer Berücksichtigung der nervösen Form. Arch. exp. Vet.-Med., 4, 44—97 (1951).

POTEL, K., und H. BINDRICH: Histologische und experimentelle Untersuchungen zur hard pad disease des Hundes unter besonderer Berücksichtigung des Encephalitis-problems. Arch. exp. Vet.-Med. 12, 897—918 (1958).

PRIDHAM, T. J., and J. BELCHER: Toxoplasmosis in mink. Canad. J. comp. Med. 22, 99—106 (1958).

PRIER, J. E., B. S. WRIGHT, and S. S. KALTER: Detection of complement-fixing antibodies for Carré's virus. Science 123, 586—587 (1965).

PRYDIE, J.: Persistence of antibodies following vaccination against canine distemper and the effect of revaccination. Vet. Rec. 78, 486—488 (1966).

PRYDIE, J. (quoted by J. GORHAM): Duration of vaccination immunity and the influence on subsequent prophylaxis. J. Amer. vet. med. Ass. 149, 699—704 (1966).

PRYDIE, J.: Resistance against canine distemper induced by measles virus. I. Measles vaccination in the presence of distemper antibodies. Vet. Rec. 83, 554—559 (1968).

PRYDIE, J., I. BATTY, and P. D. WALKER: Lack of interference in tissue culture between the viruses of canine distemper and infectious canine hepatitis as demonstrated by immunofluorescence. Vet. Rec. 79, 354 (1966).

PUNTONI, V.: Saggio di vaccinazione anticimurrosa preventiva eseguita per mezzo del virus specifico. Ann. Igiene 33, 553 (1923).

REAGAN, R. L., and A. L. BRUECKNER: Morphological studies by electron microscopy of the canine distemper virus. Cornell Vet. 41, 141—144 (1951).

Reculard, P., et J. C. Guillon: Isolement d'une souche de virus de maladie de Carré a propriétés biologique particulières. Bull. Acad. vét. Fr. **40**, 507 (1967).

Reculard, P., L. Nicol, O. Girard, R. Corvazier, M. Cheyrous et P. Sizaret: Étude du virus de Carré en cultures cellulaires. I. Culture du virus sur cellules embryonnaires de poulet. Ann. Inst. Pasteur **98**, 344—350 (1960).

Reinhard, K. R.: A distemper-like disease. Publ. Hlth Rep. (Wash.) **68**, 535—536 (1953).

Reinhard, K. R., R. L. Rausch, and R. L. Gray: Field investigations or prophylaxis against epizootic distemper in artic sled dogs. Proc. Book Amer. vet. Ass., 92 Ann. Meet., pp. 223—227 (1955).

Riazantseva, N. E.: Experimental measles in puppies. Zh. Mikrobiol. (Mosk.) **27**, 22—29 (1956).

Ribelin, W. E.: The incidence of distemper in canine encephalitis cases. Amer. J. vet. Res. **14**, 96—104 (1953).

Roberts, J. A.: A study of the relationship between human measles virus and canine distemper virus. J. Immunol. **94**, 622—628 (1965).

Robinson, V. B., J. W. Nerberne, and D. M. Brooks: Distemper in the American raccoon *(procyon lotor)*. J. Amer. vet. med. Ass. **131**, 276—278 (1957).

Robson, D. S., B. P. Hildreth, G. F. Atkinson, L. E. Carmichael, F. D. Barnes, B. Pakkola, and J. A. Baker: Standardization of quantitative serological tests. Proc. U.S. Livestock Sanit. Ass. **65**, 74—78 (1961).

Robson, D. S., R. Kenneson, J. H. Gillespie, and T. F. Benson: Statistical studies of distemper in dogs. Proc. 9th Gaines Vet. Symposium, Kankakee, Illinois **9**, 10—14 (1959).

Rockborn, G.: Viraemia and neutralizing antibodies in experimental distemper in dogs. Arch. ges. Virusforsch. **7**, 168—182 (1957 a).

Rockborn, G.: Viraemia and neutralizing antibodies in naturally acquired distemper in dogs. Arch. ges. Virusforsch. **7**, 183—190 (1957 b).

Rockborn, G.: Canine distemper virus in tissue culture. Arch. ges. Virusforsch. **8**, 485—492 (1958 a).

Rockborn, G.: Further studies on viraemia and neutralizing antibodies in naturally acquired distemper in dogs. Arch. ges. Virusforsch. **8**, 500—510 (1958 b).

Rockborn, G.: Studies över valpsjukans epizootiologi, patogenes och etiology. Institutionen för Virusforskning, Karolinska Inst., Stockholm, 1958 c.

Rockborn, G.: A study of serological immunity against distemper in an urban dog population. Arch. ges. Virusforsch. **8**, 493—499 (1958 d).

Rockborn, G.: An attenuated strain of canine distemper virus in tissue culture. Nature (Lond.) **184**, 822 (1959).

Rockborn, G.: A preliminary report on efforts to produce a living distemper vaccine in tissue culture. J. small Anim. Pract. **1**, 53 (1960).

Rockborn, G., E. Norrby, and N. Lannek: Comparison between immunizing effect in dogs and ferrets of living distemper vaccines, attenuated in dog tissue cultures and embryonated eggs. Res. vet. Sci. **6**, 423 (1965).

Röhrer, H.: Veränderungen im ZNS bei experimentell erzeugter nervöser Staupe. Arch exp. Vet.-Med. **4**, 116—118 (1951).

Rubarth, S.: An acute virus disease with liver lesion in dogs. Acta path. microbiol. scand. **69**, 1 (1947).

Rudolf, J.: Beitrag zur Staupe beim Silberfuchs, Nerz und Waschbären. Dtsch. tierärztl. Wschr. **38**, 728—732 (1930).

Sawada, M.: Pathological studies on canine distemper. I. Histopathological changes in ferrets infected with experimental canine distemper. Jap. J. vet. Sci. **27**, 121 (1965).

Scheitlin, M., E. Seiferle und H. Stünzi: Klinische und pathologisch-anatomische Beobachtungen über die sogenannte „hard-pad disease" beim Hund. Schweiz. Arch. Tierheilk. **93**, 91—129 (1951).

Schindler, R.: Bericht über das Auftreten und den Verlauf einer Staupevirusinfektion unter den Nerzen einer norddeutschen Pelztierfarm. Tierärztl. Umsch. **10**, 118—120 (1955).

SCHINDLER, R.: Untersuchungen über das Interferenzphänomen bei Staupe. Arch. ges. Virusforsch. **6**, 367—373 (1955).

SCHLINGMANN, A. S.: Studies on canine distemper. I. The bacteriology of one hundred naturally infected cases. J. Amer. vet. med. Ass. **80**, 729 (1932).

SCHÖBEL, CH.: Untersuchungen über konjunktivate Einschlußkörperchen bei Staupe. Berl. Münch. tierärztl. Wschr. **81**, 337—339 (1968).

SCHRÖDER, H.: Die Staupe des Hundes und ihre Behandlung. Buchdruckerei Gebr. Bischoff, Wittenberge, 1925.

SCHRÖDER, H. D., C. U. v. MICKWITZ und H. M. KRÄMER: Zur fluoreszenzserologischen Diagnose der Hunde-Staupe. Kleintier-Prax. **13**, 93—97 (1968).

SCHROEDER, J. P., and D. E. BORDT: Influence of amount of test virus on quantitative *in ovo* canine distemper virus neutralization test. Proc. Soc. exp. Biol. (N. Y.) **109**, 979—982 (1962).

SCHULZE, W.: Die Staupe des Hundes (vergleichende diagnostische und therapeutische Untersuchungen über die Staupe des Hundes mit besonderer Berücksichtigung der einschlägigen Literatur). Habil.-Schrift Leipzig, 1948.

SCHWARZ, A. J., P. A. BOYER, L. W. ZIRBEL, and C. J. YORK: Experimental vaccination against measles. I. Test of live measles and distemper vaccine in monkeys and 2 human volunteers under laboratory conditions. J. Amer. med. Ass. **173**, 861—867 (1960).

SCOTT, G. R., and R. D. BROWN: A neutralisation test for the detection of rinderpest antibodies. J. comp. Path. 68, 308—314 (1958).

SEDGWICK, C. J., and W. A. YOUNG: Distemper outbreak in a zoo. Mod. vet. Pract. **49**, 39 (1968).

SHAVER, D. N., R. H. BUSSELL, and A. L. BARRON: Comparative cytopathology of canine distemper and measles viruses in ferret kidney cell cultures. Arch. ges. Virusforsch. **14**, 487—498 (1964).

SHAW, R. N.: Distemper in the mink. Vet. Rec. **13**, 513—517 (1933).

SHISHIDO, A., K. YAMANOUCHI, M. HIKITA, T. SATO, A. FUKUDA, and F. KOBUNE: Development of a cell culture system susceptible to measles, canine distemper, and rinderpest viruses. Arch. ges. Virusforsch. **22**, 364—380 (1967).

SIENDENTOPF, H. A., and R. G. GREEN: Factors in the preservation of the distemper virus. J. infect. Dis. **71**, 253—259 (1942).

SIIM, J. CH., U. BIERING-SÖRENSEN, and T. MÖLLER: Toxoplasmosis in domestic animals. Advanc. vet. Sci. **8**, 335—429 (1963).

SIZARET, P., P. RECULARD et D. LABERT: Mise en évidence du virus de Carré dans des organes du furet par le test précipitation gel. Bull. Acad. vét. Fr. **63**, 119—121 (1963).

SJOLTE, I. P.: Om cytoplasmatiske og nucleare inclusioners forekomst ved spontant forekommende hyndesyge. Skand. Vet.-Tidskr. **37**, 350—364 (1947).

SKAGGS, J. W.: Canine distemper and measles. J. Amer. vet. med. Ass. **136**, 8—11 (1960).

SKALINSKI, E. I., and Y. F. BORISOVICH: Electron microscopical study of avianized canine distemper virus. Trudy nauchno Kontrol Inst. Vet. Preparatov **10**, 123—127 (1962).

SLATER, E. A.: The response to measles and distemper virus in immune-suppressed and normal dogs. J. Amer. vet. med. Ass. **156**, 1762 (1970).

SMITH, K. W.: The use of distemperoid virus. Amer. J. vet. Sci. **1**, 56 (1958).

SMITH, O. K., R. C. DUNLAP, J. F. THIEL, J. T. NEWMAN, and A. E. PALMER: Isolation of viruses from primary dog cell cultures and the occurrence of viral antibody in donor animals. Proc. Soc. exp. Biol. (N. Y.) **133**, 560—567 (1970).

SNOW, L., M. J. BURNS, and C. H. CLARK: Serum protein electrophoresis and serum transaminase activity of dogs with canine distemper. Amer. J. vet. Res. **27**, 70—73 (1966).

SOBAUGH: Cited by J. R. GORHAM: J. Amer. vet. med. Ass. **149**, 610 (1966).

SPEARMAN and KARBER (quoted by D. J. FINNEY): Statistical Method in Biological Assay. Hafner Publishing Co., New York, N. Y., 1952.

STANDFUSS, R.: Über die ätiologische und diagnostische Bedeutung der Negrischen Tollwutkörperchen. Arch. Tierheilk. **34**, 109 (1908).

STEEL, J. D., and J. H. WHITTEM: Canine distemper and distemper-like disease. Aust. vet. J. **26**, 197—212 (1950).

STEWART, D. L., C. N. HEBERT, and I. DAVIDSON: International standard for anti-canine-distemper serum. World Hlth Org. Bull. **39**, 917—924 (1968).

STONE, S. S.: Multiple components of rinderpest virus as determined by the precipitin reaction in agar gel. Virology **11**, 638—640 (1960).

STORTS, R. W., A. KOESTNER, and R. A. DENNIS: The effects of canine distemper virus on explant tissue culture of canine cerebellum. Acta neuropath. (Berl.) **11**, 1—14 (1968).

STÜNZI, H., J. H. GILLESPIE, and A. CELIKER: Pathological response of the chorio-allantoic membrane of the hen's egg to distemper virus. Cornell Vet. **44**, 211—215 (1954).

SVEHAG, S. E., and J. R. GORHAM: An attempt to demonstrate the minimal number (estimated by probit analysis) of biological units of chicken embryo-propagated distemper virus required to immunize ferrets and mink. Arch. ges. Virusforsch. **12**, 250—258 (1962).

TAJIMA, M., T. MOTOHASHI, S. KISHI, and J. NAKAMURA: A comparative electron microscopic study on the morphogenesis of canine distemper and rinderpest viruses. Jap. J. vet. Sci. **33**, 1 (1971).

TAMOGLIA, T. W.: Inactivated canine distemper virus vaccine. J. Amer. vet. med. Ass. **149**, 640—644 (1966).

THIEL, J. F., K. O. SMITH, J. NEWMAN, J. DUNN, and M. D. TROUSDALE: Isolation and identification of adventitious agents from primary cell cultures of dogs. Bact. Proc. **97**, 161 (1968).

THOMAS, E. D., J. A. BAKER, and J. W. FERREBEE: The effect of methotrexate on the production of antibodies against attenuated distemper virus in the dog. J. Immunol. **90**, 324—328 (1963).

TORNEY, H. C., D. E. BORDT, and M. THEODORE: Canine distemper immunization. Persistence of measles antibodies in dogs vaccinated with measles virus and the effect of passively transferred measles antibodies on vaccination of puppies with measles virus. Vet. Med. small Anim. Clin. **62**, 1065—1069 (1967).

TORREY, J. C., and A. H. RAHE: Studies in canine distemper. J. med. Res. **27**, 291—364 (1913).

TREVAN, D.: Discussion on some neurological diseases of man and animals. Early lesions in "nervous distemper" of dogs. Proc. roy. Soc. Med. **46**, 890—891 (1953).

VANBOGAERT, L., and J. R. M. INNES: Subacute diffuse sclerosing encephalitis in the dog. In: Comparative Neuropathology, p. 394. (INNES and SAUNDERS, eds.) Academic Press, New York, 1962.

VANTSIS, J. T.: Preliminary note on the propagation of canine distemper virus in different tissue culture systems. Vet. Rec. **71**, 99—100 (1959).

VERLINDE, J. D.: Over een nieuw type van het virus van Carré. T. Diergeneesk. **71**, 210 (1946).

VERLINDE, J. D.: Observations on types of canine encephalitis. T. Diergeneesk. **73**, 922—932 (1948).

VILLEMOT, J. A., A. PROVOST et P. GORET: Nouvelles recherches à l'immunisation croisée: Maladie de Carré-peste bovine. Rev. Élev. **14**, 233—244 (1961).

Virus Subcommittee of International Nomenclature Committee: Recommendations on virus nomenclature. Virology **21**, 516—517 (1963).

VLADIMIROV, V. V.: Haemagglutination reaction in dog distemper. Veterinariya (Moscow) **26**, (7) 59. Original not seen. Cited in Vet. Bull. **21**, 77 (1951).

WARREN, J.: The relationship of the viruses of measles, canine distemper and rinderpest. Advanc. Virus Res. **7**, 27—60 (1960).

WARREN, J., K. NADEL, E. SLATER, and S. J. MILLIAN: The canine distemper measles complex. I. Immune response of dogs to canine distemper and measles viruses. Amer. J. vet. Res. **21**, 111—119 (1960).

WATERSON, A. P.: Two kinds of myxovirus. Nature (Lond.) **193**, 1163—1164 (1962).
WATERSON, A. P., J. G. CRUIKSHANK, G. D. LAURENCE, and A. D. KANAREK: The nature of measles virus. Virology **15**, 379—382 (1961).
WATERSON, A. P., R. ROTT, and G. RUCKLE-ENDERS: The components of measles virus and their relationship to rinderpest and distemper. Z. Naturforsch. **18 b**, 377—384 (1963).
WATSON, E. A.: The use and possible effects of live virus vaccine as a means of preventing distemper on fox and mink farms. Canada, Dept. Agr., Publ. No. 649 (Cric. No. 143) (1939).
WATSON, E. A., and P. J. G. PLUMMER: Distemper inclusion bodies. Amer. J. vet. Res. **3**, 350—357 (1942).
WEST, J. L., and C. A. BRANDLY: The production of immunity to distemper in foxes by means of vaccines. Cornell Vet. **39**, 292—301 (1949).
WEST, J. L., and C. A. BRANDLY: The adaptation of fox distemper virus to white mice. Cornell Vet. **45**, 560—569 (1955).
WEST, J. L., S. H. McNUTT, and C. A. BRANDLY: The adaptation of fox distemper virus to embryonating chicken eggs. Cornell Vet. **46**, 39—50 (1956).
WHITE, G., and K. M. COWAN: Separation of the soluble antigens and infectious particles of rinderpest and canine distemper. Virology **16**, 209—211 (1962).
WHITE, G., R. M. SIMPSON, and G. R. SCOTT: An antigenic relationship between the viruses of bovine rinderpest and canine distemper. Immunology **4**, 203 (1961).
WHITNEY, L. F., and G. D. WHITNEY: The distemper complex. Pract. Sci. Publishing Co., Orange, Conn., 1953.
WHITTEM, J. H.: Recent advances in the control of animal virus diseases (with special reference to canine distemper). Aust. vet. J. **29**, 109—114 (1953).
WHITTEM, J. H., and D. C. BLOOD: Canine encephalitis: Pathological and clinical observations. Aust. vet. J. **26**, 73—83 (1950).
WINQUIST, G.: The histopathological changes of the central nervous system in canine distemper. Nord. Vet.-Med. **2**, 367—384 (1950).
WÖHLE, W.: Beziehungen zwischen Masern-, Staupe- und Rinderpestvirus. Behringwerk-Mitteilungen Heft **46**, 43 (1966).
WOODRUFF, A. M., and E. W. GOODPASTURE: The susceptibility of the chorioallantoic membrane of chick embryos to infection with the fowl-pox virus. Amer. J. Path. **7**, 209 (1931).
YAMANOUCHI, K., F. KOBUNE, A. FUKUDA, M. HAYAMI, and A. SHISHIDO: Comparative immunofluorescent studies on measles, canine distemper, and rinderpest viruses. Arch. ges. Virusforsch. **29**, 90—100 (1970).
YORK, C. J., J. L. BITTLE, G. R. BURCH, and D. E. JONES: An effective canine distemper tissue culture vaccine. Vet. Med. **55**, 30—35 (1960).
ZIMMERMANN, H.: Salmonellen als Begleitbakterien der Nerzstaupe. Mh. Vet.-Med. **17**, 306—307 (1962).
ZYDECK, F. A.: Application of the electroprecipitin test to the detection of the virus of canine distemper. Experientia (Basel) **26**, 88—90 (1970).

Marburg Virus

By

Rudolf Siegert

Hygiene Institute of the Philipps University
Pilgrimstein 2, D-355 Marburg (Lahn), Germany

With 20 Figures

Table of Contents

I. Introduction and History

Hardly any experience is more exciting for a physician than suddenly to encounter an unknown, dangerous infectious disease. In Europe no new diseases have been observed in many decades. Thus a mysterious hemorrhagic fever which broke out simultaneously in Germany and Yugoslavia in 1967 stimulated considerable interest; it posed a demanding challenge for clinicians, microbiologists, epidemiologists, and the public health service.

The disease appeared in mid-August and affected 31 persons in Marburg/Lahn, Frankfurt/Main, and Belgrade. Seven cases ended in death. At first, only employees of the Behringwerke, the Paul Ehrlich Institute and the Institute for Sera and Vaccines TORLAK became ill. All patients had had direct contact with monkeys, or with blood, organs, or tissue cultures from these animals. The common source of the infections was soon traced to certain shipments of monkeys (Cercopithecus aethiops) from Uganda. Further cases developed through contact of hospital employees with patients. In one instance, a woman contracted the disease via the semen from her husband, who had had the disease three months before.

The clinical symptoms and pathologic findings did not correspond to the picture of any known disease (MARTINI et al., 1968 a, b; STILLE et al., 1968; GEDIGK et al., 1968). The epidemiology was also unusual, considering that in spite of the use of millions of monkeys as experimental animals no such disease had ever been observed previously (HENNESSEN et al., 1968). All microbiological tests for differential diagnosis remained inconclusive, so that a new pathogenic agent had to be drawn into consideration (SIEGERT et al., 1968 b).

Of importance for the clarification of the unknown etiology was the observation, made independently in two laboratories, that guinea pigs are susceptible to the infection. After injection of patients' blood or of tissue suspensions taken during the febrile stage the animals became sick and developed a high fever (SMITH et al., 1967; SIEGERT et al., 1967 a, b; 1968 a). In the course of adaptation of the unknown agent to guinea pigs a considerable increase in virulence occurred within several passages. Reinfection of convalescent guinea pigs induced no febrile reaction, indicating the presence of an effective immunity. Neutralizing antibodies (SIEGERT et al., 1967 b; 1968 a), as well as complement-fixing antibodies with increasing titers (SMITH et al., 1967) were found in both the patients and the infected guinea pigs. Serologic cross reaction indicated that the infections in man and guinea pigs were identical. With the aid of fluorescent dye-marked immune sera from patients and experimental animals, cytoplasmic inclusions were demonstrated in tissue preparations from affected guinea pigs and patients, as well as in infected cell cultures (SIEGERT et al., 1967 b; 1968 b, c; SLENCZKA et al., 1968).

Experimental transmission of the unknown agent to Cercopithecus monkeys using blood taken from patients and guinea pigs during the febrile stage confirmed the high infectivity and pathogenicity for monkeys. Comparative histopathology revealed the tissue damage to be of substantially similar nature in man, guinea pigs, and monkeys (SMITH et al., 1967; GEDIGK et al., 1968; SIMPSON et al., 1968 a, b; HAAS et al., 1968 a, b; BECHTELSHEIMER, 1968).

Two different opinions existed initially concerning the nature of the pathogenic agent. The Porton team in England (SMITH et al., 1967; SIMPSON, 1969 c; ZLOTNIK et al., 1968 a) considered the cytoplasmic granula which they observed by light microscopy in livers of infected guinea pigs and in cell cultures to be rickettsia or organisms of the psittacosis-lymphogranuloma group. This assumption seemed to be supported by the size, shape, and staining qualities of the granula, as well as the pathogenicity of the agent for guinea pigs and its failure to grow in artificial nutrient media.

In contrast, SIEGERT et al. (1967 a, b) suggested a viral agent because of the submicroscopic size, the cell-dependent replication, and the cytoplasmic antigen inclusions. Only electron microscopy could be expected to reveal the actual nature of the pathogen. Following systematic enrichment by means of several passages in guinea pigs, it was possible to demonstrate directly a strandlike virus of unusual length in plasma, liver, and spleen of the infected animals. The same agent was found electron microscopically in patients' blood during the febrile stage, as well as in experimentally infected monkeys and cell cultures (SIEGERT et al., 1967 a, b; PETERS and MÜLLER, 1968). The complex structure of the new virus, which was provisionally named the "Marburg virus", suggested its possible relatedness to the vesicular stomatitis and rabies viruses. These results were soon corroborated by other research teams. In spite of intensive efforts, however, it has not yet been possible to trace the origin and the natural reservoir of the "Marburg virus" (SLENCZKA et al., 1971).

II. Classification and Nomenclature

There can be no doubt that the pathogen responsible for the "Marburg monkey disease" fulfills the morphologic and biologic criteria for a virus. This is indicated by its cell-dependent replication, as well as its complex structure and helical symmetry. The genetic material is RNA.

Most authors agree that the structural pattern of the "Marburg virus" (Figs. 1—4) exhibits many features similar to that of the vesicular stomatitis and rabies viruses (SIEGERT et al., 1967 a, b; PETERS and MÜLLER, 1968; KUNZ et al., 1968 a; HAAS et al., 1968 b; KISSLING et al., 1968; MAY et al., 1968; ZLOTNIK and SIMPSON, 1968). Although there are several different group names for these viruses, rhabdoviruses is the one most commonly used (MELNICK and McCOMBS, 1966). This group includes the Egtved virus of rainbow trout, cocal virus, sigma virus of Drosophila, the Flanders Hart Park and Kern Canyon viruses, and various plant viruses (ZWILLENBERG et al., 1965; PETERS et al., 1971).

According to PETERS et al. (1971), the most important common features include the existence of two transverse striation patterns of different periodicity, spike-like projections on the surface of the envelope, bead-string-like substructures of the nucleocapsid, and occasional branching (p. 104). There is likewise some similarity in the morphogenesis and in the structure of the cytoplasmic inclusions (p. 120).

The coiled and circular forms characteristic of the Marburg virus have occasionally been observed in rhabdoviruses. PETERS and MÜLLER (1968), as well as

PETERS et al. (1971), consider the unusual pleomorphism and length of the virus, which is about three times as long as the rhabdoviruses, not to be of such fundamental importance as to exclude it from this group. ALMEIDA et al. (1971), on the other hand, do not share this point of view, but regard these differences between the Marburg virus and the rhabdovirus group as essential. MAY and HERZBERG (1969) do not dispute a relatedness, but point out certain differences with respect to the vesicular stomatitis virus. These include size, form, the behavior in cell cultures, and the photodynamic sensitivity of the Marburg virus to methylene blue. They suggest that these properties should be drawn into consideration in determining the definitive classification. MURPHY et al. (1971) point out several differences with respect to structural properties of the virus particles and the morphogenesis compared with established taxonomic schema so that the Marburg virus should still remain unclassified.

A few arboviruses are included in the rhabdovirus group; the arbovirus category is based on ecological criteria. The assignment of the Marburg virus to this group is supported by its sensitivity to ether and deoxycholate (SIEGERT et al., 1968 a; KUNZ et al., 1968 a), its capability of multiplication in baby mouse brains (Kunz et al., 1968 a; HOFMANN and KUNZ, 1970), and its replication in the thorax of Aedes aegypti (KUNZ et al., 1968 b; HOFMANN et al., 1969). It has not yet been proved, however, that the Marburg virus can be transmitted by arthropods. The fact that no antigenic relatedness to the arboviruses has been found (CASALS, 1967; 1971) still does not exclude it from this group. Although a few questions remain to be answered, application has already been made to include the Marburg virus in the catalogue of the arthropod-borne viruses of the world (SIMPSON, 1969 a).

With respect to the classification an interesting report was published by ALMEIDA et al. (1969), who observed that the Marburg virus bore a striking morphologic similarity to tubular structures regularly found in Leptospira cultures. It has not been clarified whether these structures represent stages in the life cycle of Leptospira, some kind of bacteriophage, or artifacts. It was suggested that the Marburg virus might be an aberrant form of Leptospira wich has become adapted to animal cells without reverting to a free-living form. It is known, however, that Leptospira structures lack the inner helix of the Marburg virus (ALMEIDA et al., 1971). The two therefore cannot be so closely related as was initially speculated. The assumption of a relatedness no longer seems valid in view of the clear differences found by PETERS et al. (1969 a) in distribution of length, form, and in ultrastructure, especially the periodicity of the striations.

Various suggestions concerning nomenclature have been made. The original, provisional name of "Marburg virus" (SIEGERT et al., 1967 b), however, has prevailed. It was initially chosen because the pathogen was first isolated from patients in Marburg. The name "vervet monkey disease agent" is also found ZLOTNIK et al., 1968 b). Rhabdovirus simiae has been proposed as a systematic name (KUNZ et al., 1968). MAY and HERZBERG (1969) suggest that the term "hamatum" or "tubulo-hamatum" should follow the group name, in order to emphasize the peculiar form (e. g., rhabdo- or arbovirus simiae hamatum or tubulo-hamatum). ALMEIDA et al. (1971) consider the Marburg virus a representative of a new group of viruses, which they refer to as "toroviruses" (p. 103).

III. Properties of the Virus

A. Morphology

1. Shape

The morphology of the Marburg virus is unusual, and is characterized by pleomorphic filaments of exceptional length (Figs. 1—4). Besides straight rods, numerous particles are found which are bent into horseshoes or 6's as well as hooks and loops. The ends are rounded; in some cases one pole is dilated, and occasional

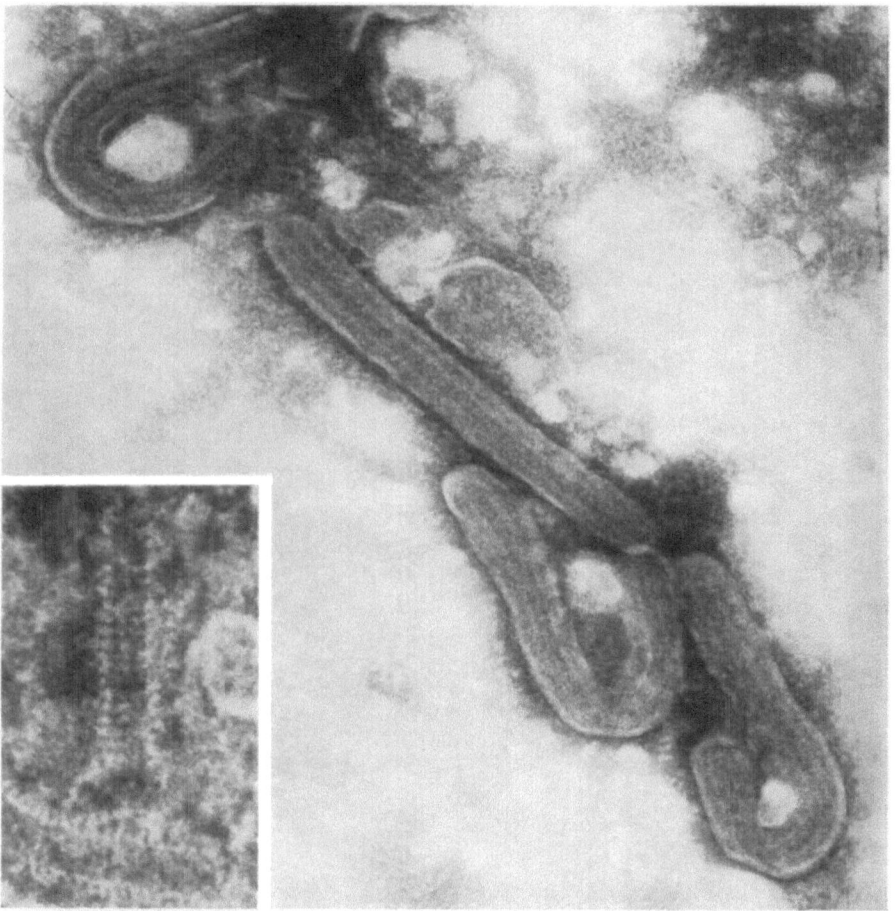

Fig. 1. Electron micrograph of Marburg virus pelleted from infectious guinea pig blood. One straight and three coiled virus particles of similar length with cross striations and axial core are seen. Glutar- and formaldehyde; negative staining (× 100,000). Insertion: naked nucleocapsid (× 300,000). Courtesy Prof. PETERS and Dr. MÜLLER, Hamburg

branching is seen. The particles were found in blood and organ tissues of patients and of experimentally infected animals, as well as in cell cultures (SIEGERT et al., 1967 a, b; KUNZ et al., 1968 a; PETERS and MÜLLER, 1968; HAAS et al., 1968 b; KISSLING et al., 1968; SMITH, 1968; MAY et al., 1968; ZLOTNIK et al., 1968 b; BOWEN et al., 1969; STOJKOVIĆ et al., 1971).

ALMEIDA *et al.* (1971) distinguish three basic forms: (1) a naked helix, and (2) coiled structures enclosed by a membrane, both of which are considered "immature", in contrast to (3) a circular, presumably "mature" form. To the last they

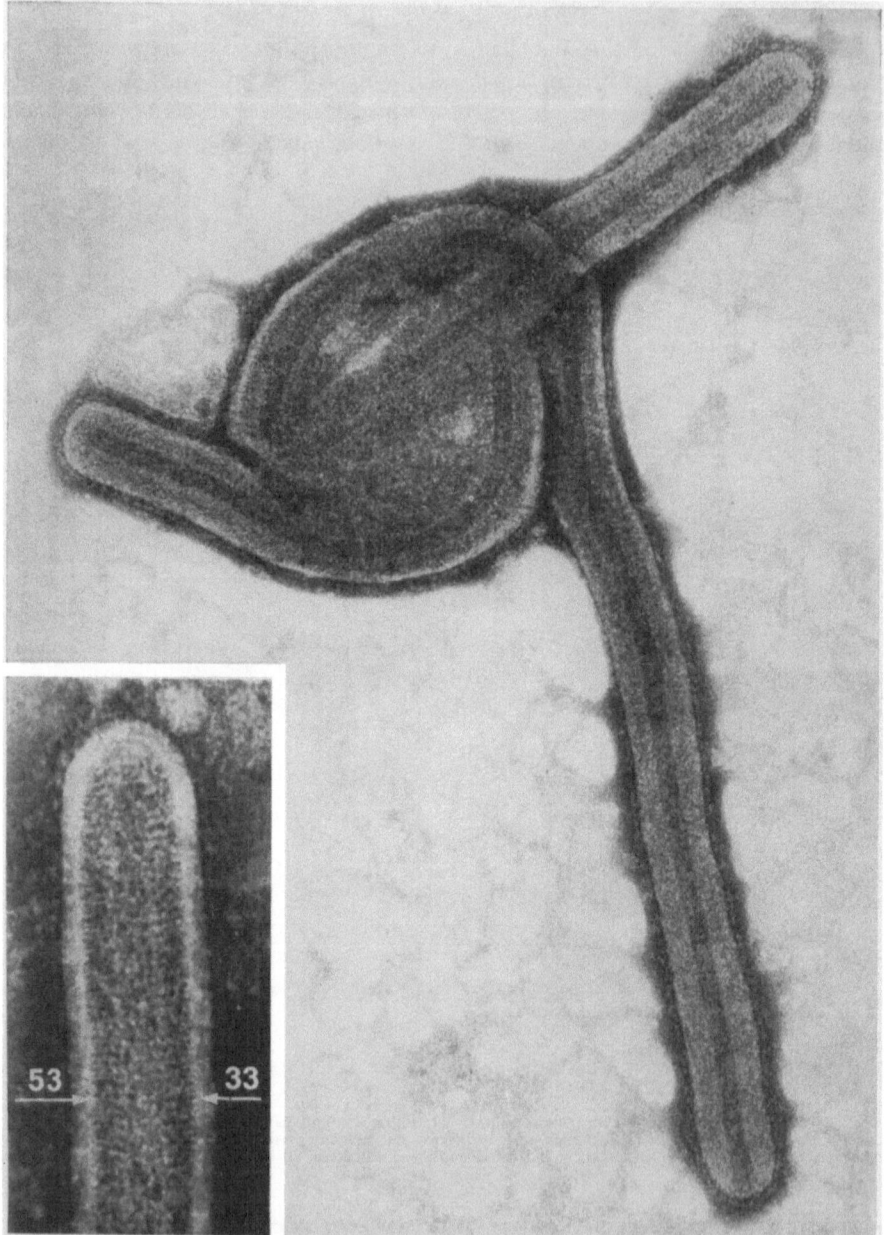

Fig. 2. Electron micrograph showing a virus particle about 2 µ long, *i. e.*, three times the normal length, together with a normal particle. The bend in the long particle divides it into ⅓ and ⅔. The central axis is clearly visible, and the cross striations are recognizable in certain portions. Superficial projections ("spikes") are evident on the exposed surfaces of the particles. Preparation as in Fig. 1 (× 140,000). Courtesy Prof. PETERS and Dr. MÜLLER, Hamburg. Insertion: Terminal portion of a particle, showing the internal, coarse cross striations with a periodicity of about 53 Å, as well as the external, finer cross striations of about 33 Å periodicity (× 290,000)

have applied the geometrical term "torus". Intermediate forms have also been described. The virus specificity of the particles was demonstrated by their capacity for binding conjugated antibodies, as seen in immunoelectron microscopy. Corresponding structures were also found by PETERS *et al.* (1971), whereas MAY and HERZBERG (1969) described coiled and circular forms, but did not observe any free helices.

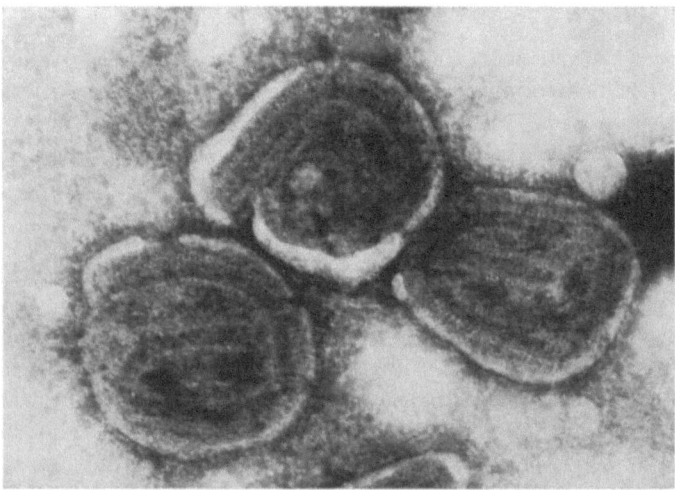

Fig. 3. Electron micrograph of three circular forms of the Marburg virus. The concave portion of the nucleocapsid is often naked. Preparation as in Fig. 1 (× 140,000). Courtesy Prof. PETERS and Dr. MÜLLER, Hamburg

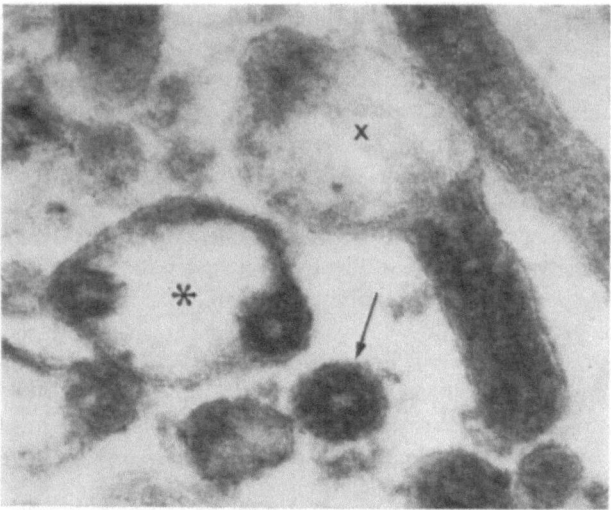

Fig. 4. Electron micrograph of Marburg virus particles in a guinea pig liver cell, four days after infection. Arrow: transverse section of a virus particle with lucent axis and double-layered envelope; asterisk: section through a coiled strand, entirely enclosed by the envelope; X: longitudinal section through a virus particle with a clublike end (artifact?) and 53 Å cross striation at the opposite end. Glutar- and formaldehyde and OsO$_4$ fixation; embedding in Durcopan; UO$_2$-acetate and Pb-citrate stain (× 170,000). Courtesy Prof. PETERS and Dr. MÜLLER, Hamburg

2. Size

Various authors are in close agreement in their size determinations of the Marburg virus by electron microscopy. The mean length, which varies considerably, is 665 mμ. About ten per cent of the particles were longer than 900 mμ; some exhibited the extreme length of 1200 mμ. The cross-sectional diameter was between 70 and 80 mμ (PETERS and MÜLLER, 1968; 1969 a; PETERS et al., 1971; HÜLSER, 1968). The circular forms have a diameter of 300—400 mμ (ALMEIDA et al., 1971).

Size determinations using filters of different pore diameter were less accurate because of the pleomorphism and variable length of the virus particles. They indicated dimensions between approximately 450 and 1000 mμ (SMITH et al., 1967; MAY and KNOTHE, 1968). For safe elimination of the infectious agent by filtration a pore size of 100 mμ or less is needed (BOWEN et al., 1969).

3. Ultrastructure

Electron microscopy of negatively stained ultra-thin sections (Figs. 1—4) revealed a complex, highly regular internal structure of the virions (PETERS and MÜLLER, 1968; 1969 b; PETERS et al., 1971), involving an envelope of about 20 mμ thickness which is covering a cylindric structure with a diameter of approximately 30 mμ. The cylindric structure, which is considered the nucleocapsid, exhibits clear transversal striations having a periodicity of about 53 Å, and a more darkly stained central axis about 20 mμ in diameter. The striations are regarded as evidence of a helical formation. The ends of ring-shaped particles apparently do not merge, even if they touch. The nucleocapsid usually consists of a single strand. Breaks in the nucleo capsid are generally found in the coiled portion; they are probably artifacts. Filaments of extreme length frequently exhibit parts lacking a nucleocapsid. Very rarely, branched particles are found. The envelope of these particles divides without interruption in three directions. It is not yet clear, however, whether the nucleocapsid also branches.

The envelope consists of several layers. The outer layer is approximately 100 Å thick; the surface is covered with spikes around 70 Å long, which are placed about 100 Å apart. The second layer is referred to as the "intermediate layer". It may exhibit cross striations of shorter periodicity (about 33 Å). The nucleocapsid may also be found without any envelope.

Further details of the structure of the Marburg virus are presented in a study by ALMEIDA et al. (1971). These authors expand their observations on morphology into speculative hypotheses concerning function. The naked helix has a linear structure of varying length (50—80 mμ). Other characteristics, such as the central core with a diameter of 28 mμ, are constant. The coiled particles are especially pleomorphic, and are described as "enveloped", "full", or "empty".

The membranes of the "enveloped" particles exhibit projections about 10mμ in length. No other distinct structures were clearly discernable. The diameter of these particles was between 72 and 110 mμ.

The "full" particles are thought to be capable of replication, and are referred to as "mature". The outer likewise shows projections and lacks a regular structure. It is similar to the envelope of many viruses, and encloses the inner helix with the central core.

The "empty" particles show no internal structure, and are smaller than the coiled particles. They are referred to as "incomplete", because they contain no inner helix. Probably they correspond to the portions of empty envelopes described by PETERS et al. (1971).

The "mature" particles are arranged like and probably develop from the "full", coiled structures. Usually they are ring-shaped (torus), but open rings and bretzel configurations have also been observed. A noteworthy feature of the ring forms is the varying number of constrictions. The breaks in the helix which correspond to these constrictions are most likely artifacts. Although the number varied, each ring usually contained four helix fragments. Occasionally the envelope surrounded the entire structure, giving it the appearance of a nearly biconcave disc. Exposure to 4° and 37° C resulted in a progressive rounding of the virions to spheres, but not into subunits (HÜLSER, 1969).

B. Physicochemical Structure

The physicochemical composition of the Marburg virus is still largely unknown. Only a small amount of indirect information is available. Experiments involving metabolic inhibitors or chemical-enzymatic inactivation experiments and cytochemical techniques on infected cells indicate that the genetic material is RNA. Replication of the virus in cell cultures could not be inhibited by either 5-iodo- or bromodeoxyuridine (40 µg/ml) (SHU et al., 1968; KISSLING et al., 1968; SLENCZKA, 1969 a; HÜLSER, 1969; BOWEN et al., 1969), or by actinomycin D (1 µg/ml) (SLENCZKA et al., 1969 a, b; MALHERBE and STRICKLAND-CHOLMLEY,1971). These findings have received further support from ultracytochemical studies. Using HCl-silver-methenamine, DNA could be demonstrated neither in virus particles of various developmental stages nor in inclusions of infected cells (PETERS et al., 1971).

Results of chemical analyses of purified virus suspensions are not yet available. Preliminary experiments with lipid solvents and enzymes provide evidence that the infectious virus particles contain lipoprotein (p. 110). The nature of the ultrastructure also suggests the presence of lipid in the envelope (ALMEIDA et al., 1971).

Hemagglutinins and hemolysins could not be demonstrated in virus-containing blood serum (10^5 ID_{50}/ml), nor in the supernatant of infected cell cultures or homogenized cell suspensions, using erythrocytes from chicken, goose, guinea pig, or man (SIEGERT and SHU, 1967/1968; MALHERBE and STRICKLAND-CHOLMLEY, 1971). Nevertheless, these negative findings do not provide conclusive proof of the absence of hemagglutinins and hemolysins. The studies must be repeated with more purified and higher concentrated virus suspensions. The hemadsorption phenomenon was not observed by any of the authors cited.

C. Antigenic Properties

1. Immunofluorescence

Using COONS' direct immunofluorescence technique, virus specific antigen was first demonstrated in cytoplasmic inclusions in histologic preparations from patients and experimentally infected animals and in cell cultures (SIEGERT et al.,

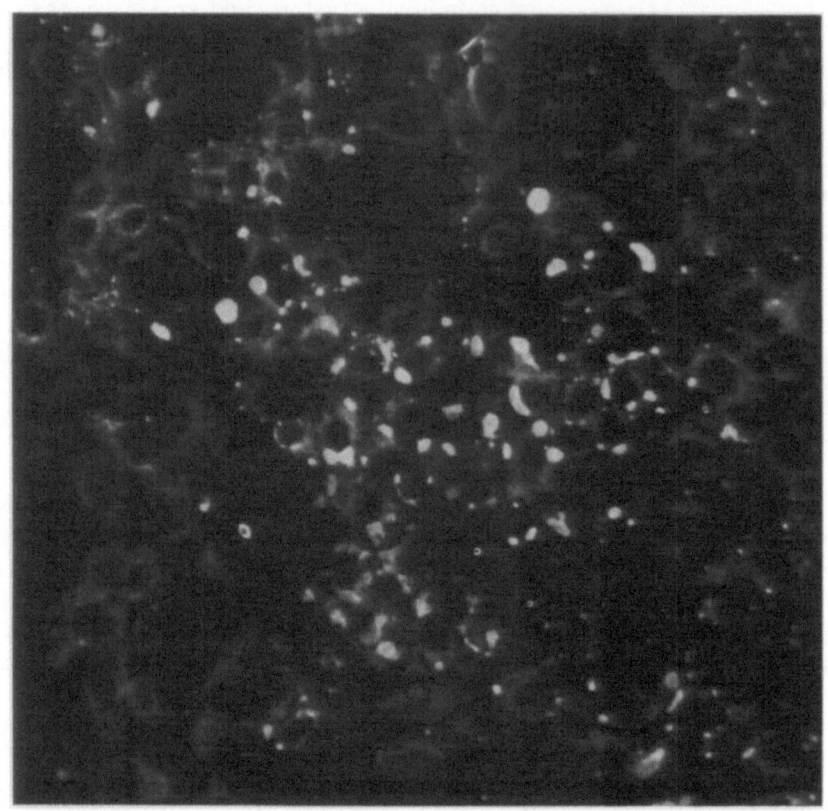

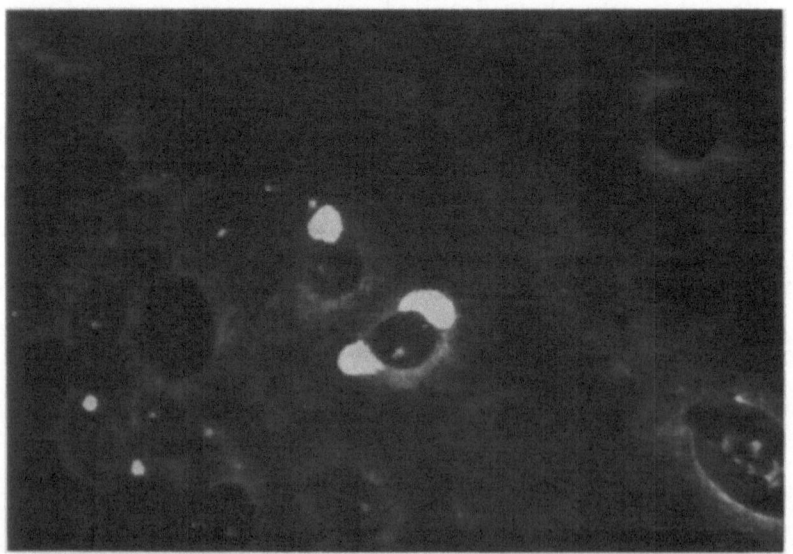

Fig. 5 a–c. Demonstration of viral antigen by direct immunofluorescence in Vero cells four days after infection with Marburg virus of the sixth passage. a) × 128, b) × 320, c) × 800. Courtesy Dr. SLENCZKA, Marburg

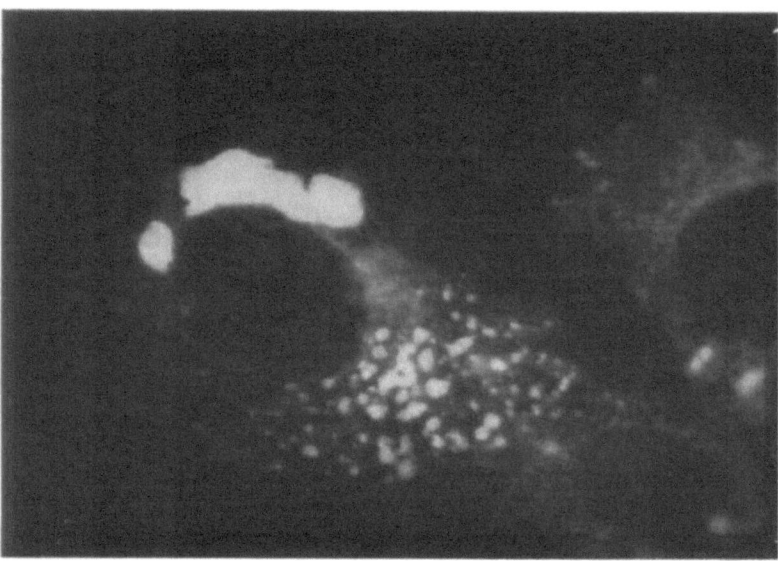

Fig. 5 c

1967 b, 1968 c; SLENCZKA *et al.*, 1968; HAAS *et al.*, 1968 b; CARTER and BRIGHT, 1968; MAASS *et al.*, 1969; HOFMANN and KUNZ, 1971).

The antigen inclusions (Figs. 5 a–c) vary in shape (spheres, dumbbells, bands, and spirals) and size (1–5 μ, occasionally up to 10 μ). In some cases the antigen is dispersed as fine granula in the cytoplasm. Accumulations of antigen can also be identified with the phase contrast microscope (SIEGERT *et al.*, 1967 b, 1968 b; SLENCZKA *et al.*, 1968). They can be stained with methylene blue-fuchsin using the method of SELLERS (SLENCZKA, 1969 a, b). The ultrastructure of the inclusions is discussed elsewhere (p. 125). As previously stated, the antigen activity of individual virus particles has been conclusively shown by immunoelectron microscopy (ALMEIDA *et al.*, 1971).

2. Neutralization

The initial source of antigen for neutralization experiments was blood of infected patients and guinea pigs. 10^2–10^3 ID_{50} of antigen were combined with antiserum and incubated for 2 hours at 37° C. The mixture was then injected intraperitoneally into guinea pigs. Inhibition of the febrile reaction was the parameter of the neutralizing effect of the antiserum (SIEGERT *et al.*, 1968 a).

Neutralization experiments using cell cultures were unsatisfactory, because the Marburg virus induces only an incomplete cytopathic effect (CPE), or none at all (p. 126). A relatively clear CPE could be obtained in the AH-1 line (green monkey kidney) which was used by HENDERSON *et al.* (1971) in neutralization tests. They incubated 30–300 $TCID_{50}$/0.1 ml for one hour at 37° C with antiserum before adding the mixture to the indicator cultures. A distinct CPE can be observed in Vero cells after several passages of the virus. This system, however, is not useful as an indicator for neutralization either; in spite of the replication of the virus, development of the CPE is inhibited by normal human serum in the medium

in concentrations as low as 5–10 per cent (SLENCZKA and WOLFF, 1971). Therefore, the percentage of cells showing cytoplasmic inclusions in the presence of
antiserum and normal serum, respectively, was used as a parameter for the neutralization effect (SLENCZKA, 1969 a, b). This method is comparable in principle
to the plaque reduction technique. In contrast to usual neutralization procedures,
high doses of infectious material (about 10^5 $TCID_{50}$/ml) are necessary to induce
cytoplasmic inclusions in more than 80 per cent of the cells within 60 hours post
infection. Counting was carried out after staining by SELLERS' method, or with
the aid of direct immunofluorescence. This procedure is also not very well suited
for routine use.

3. Complement Fixation

Antigens for the demonstration of complement-fixing (CF) antibodies were
usually prepared from cell-free organ extracts from experimentally infected animals. Comparison of the following experiments was not possible, because in most
cases, the authors did not provide data on the virus concentration or appropriate
controls. The antigen used by SMITH et al. (1967) and STOJKOVIĆ et al. (1971) was
an aqueous extract of guinea pig spleen treated with 2 per cent chloroform and
containing merthiolate (1 : 10,000). SIMPSON et al. (1968 a) carried out their
experiments with 20 per cent suspensions of guinea pig liver or spleen or vervet
monkey liver after treatment with 0.5 per cent formalin and several ether ex-
tractions. KISSLING et al. (1968) also used 20 per cent suspensions of guinea pig
liver; however, they added β-propiolactone (1 : 2000) to reduce the infectivity of
the antigen. KALTER et al. (1969) and KALTER (1971) have reported experiments
with the same antigen. HOFMANN and KUNZ (1969 a) described studies with an
antigen from virus-infected guinea pig liver in the ninth passage. They took
advantage of the observation that the virus accumulates with each passage. In
later experiments HOFMANN and KUNZ (1970) used an antigen from the brains of
mice which had been infected with a neuro-adapted strain of the virus. The tests
of HENDERSON et al. (1971) were carried out with an antigen partially purified by
absorption with hamster liver powder. The antigen used by STRICKLAND-CHOLM-
LEY and MALHERBE (1970, 1971) consisted of a 20 per cent suspension of monkey
liver or spleen. The liver antigen had a titer of 10^3 $TCID_{50}$/ml. The preparations
were treated with fluorocarbon in order to remove nonspecific components.
It was reported that inactivation of the infectivity (e. g., by heating to 56° C or
by treatment with β-propiolactone) can reduce the antigen titer (KISSLING et al.,
1968; HOFMANN and KUNZ, 1969 a). Antigen preparations from organ suspensions contain variable amounts of nonspecific components (STRICKLAND-CHOLMLEY
and MALHERBE, 1970; SLENCZKA and WOLFF, 1971; SLENCZKA et al., 1970, 1971).

Antigens prepared from infected cell cultures have the advantage of being
more specific. "Chronically" infected Vero carrier cultures have proved valuable
because they contain a sufficient amount (10^6 $TCID_{50}$/ml) of virus (SLENCZKA
et al., 1970). The antigen was twice as effective after ether extraction. Indirect
immunofluorescence proved to be more sensitive than the CF test for antibody
assays. Antigen preparations from chronically infected BHK-21 cells were also
used (SLENCZKA et al., 1971). MALHERBE and STRICKLAND-CHOLMLEY (1971) did not
succeed in obtaining complement-fixing antigen from infected vervet monkey

kidney monolayer cultures or from flask cultures of minced monkey liver or spleen.

The antigen activity of the Marburg virus is intimately associated with the virus particles; there is no evidence for the existence of soluble antigen. The virus strains tested were serologically uniform. The physicochemical nature of the antigen has not yet been characterized on purified virus suspensions, nor has the correlation between the antigen structure, virus replication, and intracellular structures been studied. Further experiments are necessary to determine the stability of the antigen under various storage conditions, and methods have to be found to inactivate the infectivity of the virus without reducing the antigen activity.

Systematic comparative studies of antibody assays are not available; it is therefore not possible to decide which procedure is most sensitive. Patient sera showing a peak titer of 1 : 64 in CF tests exhibited a poor activity in neutralization tests using guinea pigs as an indicator system (HOFMANN and KUNZ, 1968). The discrepancy was probably due to nonspecific components contaminating the complement-fixing antigen preparation from organ material. Neutralization tests using cell cultures derived from green monkey kidney (AH₁ strain), on the other hand, were more frequently positive than CF reactions with inactivated antigen from guinea pig liver (HENDERSON et al., 1971). Antibody assays by agar gel precipitation were not successful (STOJKOVIĆ et al., 1971). The antigen used, however, was only a roughly purified suspension of liver tissue from experimentally infected guinea pigs. The virus titer of the suspension was not mentioned.

4. Immune Sera

The immune sera for antigen activity tests were derived from patients and experimentally infected guinea pigs. The animals used had survived the first infection of the Marburg virus and had been repeatedly reinfected (SMITH et al., 1967; SIEGERT et al., 1968 a; HOFMANN and KUNZ, 1969 a). In order to obtain a sufficient antibody titer, KISSLING et al. (1968) recommended injection of a 20 per cent suspension of inactivated liver tissue into the guinea pigs two weeks prior to infection with the fully virulent agent. They reduced the infectivity of the liver tissue suspension by exposure to β-propiolactone for 24 hours. This pretreatment nevertheless did not protect guinea pigs or monkeys against subsequent infection with fully virulent virus. As a result only one immune serum from a moribund monkey could be obtained in this way (MALHERBE and STRICKLAND-CHOLMLEY, 1971). Hyperimmune sera from animals generally had maximum titers which were one dilution step above those of the patients.

5. Serologic Cross Reactions

The Marburg virus seems to have unique antigen properties. No serological relatedness was found to any of approximately 200 microorganisms and viruses tested. Detailed comparative studies have been carried out with arboviruses, especially those of the VSV group (CASALS, 1967, 1971; SMITH et al., 1967; KUNZ et al., 1968 a; KISSLING et al., 1968). Arbovirus antigen preparations and immune sera from patients and guinea pigs infected with Marburg virus were tested in CF and hemagglutination inhibition reactions to examine the serologic relatedness.

The combination Marburg virus antigen – arbovirus immune sera was used in only a few cases. In spite of similarity in morphology between the Marburg virus and the rabies virus and of their respective cytoplasmic inclusions, no antigen relatedness was evident in studies involving CF tests and immunization experiments of infected animals. In direct immunofluorescence, Negri bodies of rabies virus in infected BHK cells could be stained with conjugated antibodies against Marburg virus. Conversely, Marburg virus-induced inclusions in Vero cells could not be stained with conjugated rabies antiserum (SLENCZKA and WOLFF, 1971).

D. Resistance to Physical and Chemical Treatment

There are discrepancies in reports concerning the effect of physical (e. g., kinetics of heat inactivation) and chemical treatment of the Marburg virus. This is not unexpected, because the experiments were not carried out with purified virus preparations. The studies were performed primarily for safety reasons, to reduce the danger in handling the antigen during serologic and histologic investigations. Attempts were also made to find appropriate chemotherapy against the virus.

The infectivity of the Marburg virus in blood plasma was destroyed within 30 minutes at 60° C (SIEGERT, 1967), and the antigen activity of a cell-free culture fluid was considerably reduced after 30 minutes at 56° C (KISSLING et al., 1968). BOWEN et al. (1969) studied the heat inactivation of the infectivity in more detail. Complete inactivation of a 10 per cent suspension of infected monkey liver (10^6 ID_{50} for guinea pigs/0.1 ml) was obtained only after 60 minutes at 56° C.

MALHERBE and STRICKLAND-CHOLMLEY (1971) found a small amount of heat resistant virus after heating of a cell-free suspension for 30 minutes at 56° C and for 10 minutes at 60° C. Heating for 20 minutes at 60° C, however, eliminated the infectivity. 0.05 M magnesium chloride did not protect the virus from heat in-activation (1 hour at 50° C).

UV irradiation inactivated the infectivity of the virus within 0.5 to 2 minutes (BOWEN et al., 1969; MALHERBE and STRICKLAND-CHOLMLEY, 1971). Inactivation resulting from a photodynamic effect occurred within 30 seconds with methylene blue or thiopyronine (MAY and HERZBERG, 1969). Virus which had been cultured in the presence of neutral red lost its infectivity after exposure to light (SLENCZKA, 1968).

Storage of a highly infectious 10 per cent suspension of liver tissue at room temperature or 4° C for five weeks resulted in only a slight decrease of the virus titer; after eight weeks the titer was markedly reduced. There was no loss of infectivity after storage for one year at − 70° C (BOWEN et al., 1969).

The Marburg virus is sensitive to ether, chloroform, and deoxycholate (SIEGERT et al., 1968 a; KUNZ et al., 1968 a; KISSLING et al., 1968; BOWEN et al., 1969; MALHERBE and STRICKLAND-CHOLMLEY, 1971). Treatment with trypsin reduced the virus titer of supernatants of cell cultures and of liver tissue suspensions (SLENCZKA, 1968; BOWEN et al., 1969).

The infectivity of the virus in liver tissue suspensions was destroyed within one hour at room temperature by exposure to 1 per cent formaldehyde, 90 per cent acetone, 2 per cent chloros, 90 per cent methyl alcohol, and Tego MGH. Fixation with osmium tetroxide inactivated the infectivity within 24 hours. The inactivating effect of 0.5 per cent carbolic acid and 2 per cent cetramide was incomplete (Bowen et al., 1969). Aluminium chloride (0.2 mM) added to monkey kidney cell culture media in order to eliminate the activity of various other agents was ineffective against the Marburg virus (MALHERBE and STRICKLAND-CHOLMLEY, 1971).

SMITH et al. (1967) and BOWEN et al. (1969) studied the inhibitory effect of antibiotics (tetracyclines and chloramphenicol) and sulfonamides (sulfamezathine, gantrisin) on replication of the virus in experimentally infected tissue cultures and guinea pigs, as well as the direct action on the virus in vitro. No evidence for a therapeutic effect was found. Clinical observations support these results.

E. Experimental Hosts and Cultivation

1. Host-Cell Range

a) Monkey

All experimental infections of monkeys (Cercopithecus aethiops, Macaca mulatta, Saimiri sciureus) were fatal, even when the infectious doses were extremely small. Only in an experimental series of MURPHY et al. (1971) one monkey did not show any signs of virus multiplication by day 6 postinfection. The animals were inoculated in various ways (subcutaneously, nasopharyngeally, intraperitoneally, and intracerebrally) with blood samples or organ suspensions from patients, experimentally infected monkeys, guinea pigs, or hamsters, or with cell culture material (SMITH et al., 1967; HAAS et al., 1968 a, b; 1969; HAAS and MAASS, 1971; SIMPSON et al., 1968 a, b; SIMPSON, 1969 b, d; MALHERBE and STRICKLAND-CHOLMLEY, 1971).

The symptoms of the monkey disease have been described by SIMPSON et al. (1968 a, b), SIMPSON (1969 b, d), and HAAS et al. (1968 a, b). The incubation period lasted from 1 to 6 days (in cases with small infectious doses up to 10 days). Following subcutaneous inoculation it was clearly longer than after intraperitoneal infection. The symptoms were generally few and nonspecific. As a rule, fever exceeding 40° C was observed, along with alterations in the blood picture. The number of granulocytes was markedly decreased. After a brief rise, the lymphocyte count dropped, in some cases to as little as 10 per cent of the initial count. The hematocrit decreased 5 to 6 per cent in the first few days; in addition, thrombocyte depletion with a reduction of the normal count by 50 to 80 per cent occurred, although the clotting time was usually not substantially extended. Basophilic granula (0.2–0.4 μ) appeared in the monocytoid cells; their frequency increased as the disease progressed. Loss of weight due to anorexia was evident; nevertheless, only in the last 1 or 2 days prior to death did the animals appear ill. The most remarkable symptom, observed only in a few rhesus monkeys, consisted of a petechial rash on the thighs, the flexor side of the arms, and less frequently on the face and upper thorax (SIMPSON et al., 1968 a, b; SIMPSON, 1969 b, d). Vaginal or rectal bleeding occurred in a few animals in terminal stages; in one case tarry stools were observed. Two monkeys had diarrhea. Blood taken from moribund monkeys often failed to clot. Thus, many of the findings were in agreement with, those observed on the patients. The interval between the time of infection and death varied from 5 to 25 days, according to the infectious dose.

During the febrile phase unusually high concentrations of virus were found in blood and organ suspensions. Even when diluted $1 : 10^{-10}$, this material was infectious for monkeys (HAAS et al., 1968 b; SIMPSON, 1969 b). Some urine and saliva samples still proved capable of infecting guinea pigs at dilutions of $1 : 10^{-3}$ to $1 : 10^{-6}$ (SIMPSON et al., 1968 a). These findings are of great epidemiologic significance, for they suggest that, in addition to contact infection, air-borne transmission to man and monkeys is also possible. The high concentration of virus in blood, organs, and products of excretion permits direct electron microscopic demonstration of the virus (PETERS and MÜLLER, 1968; HAAS et al., 1968 b; BOWEN et al., 1969), as well as direct demonstration of antigen by means of immunofluorescence (HAAS et al., 1968 b; MAASS et al., 1969; HAAS and MAASS, 1971). BOWEN et al. (1969) found it noteworthy that they were unable to find the long, membranous "bulbous heads" of the pathogen in monkey plasma which ZLOTNIK et al. (1968 b) had observed in organ tissues.

Pathologic-anatomic changes in the monkeys were often complicated to a varying extent by preexisting diseases. Nevertheless, the rest of the findings were uniform and can be regarded on the basis of comparative pathology as being due to the virus (SIMPSON et al., 1968 b; HAAS et al., 1968 a; ZLOTNIK, 1969; OEHLERT, 1971).

Macroscopically, the lungs, liver, and spleen of many rhesus monkeys exhibited tuberculous caseation; in the cercopithecans hemorrhagic, suppurative pneumonia was most striking. The spleens were enlarged, soft, and brittle. Both monkey species exhibited pulmonary, hepatic, and splenic parenchymal bleedings, and enlargement and fatty change in the liver.

Microscopic examination revealed tuberculous changes, malaria, filiariasis, and worm infections. It is impossible to estimate the extent to which the deaths of the animals were attributable to these accompanying infections.

Definitely caused by the virus were the necroses involving single cells and small cell groups in the liver, with perifocal hemorrhages, glycogen depletion of the parenchyma, and fatty degeneration. No inflammatory response was observed.

Follicular necroses, perifollicular bleeding, and reduction in the number of cells in the red pulp were found in the spleen and lymph nodes. Higher magnification revealed necrosis of most of the reticular cells, which amassed in places to form homogeneous clumps of debris. The interspaces contained deposits of fibrin and platelets.

In the cytoplasm of the liver, spleen, and lymph nodes eosinophilic, Feulgen-negative inclusions were found, the number of which increased with the duration of the illness. Their formation marked the beginning of a process leading to necrosis. It seems likely that these inclusions are identical with those revealed by immuno-fluorescence (HAAS et al., 1968 a, b). The intracytoplasmic basophilic bodies (vervet monkey disease = VDM bodies) observed in guinea pigs could not be found in monkeys (ZLOTNIK, 1969). It is doubtful whether they correspond to the structures described by HAAS et al. (1968 a, b). The VMD bodies must be differentiated from various basophilic, Feulgen-positive inclusions, which probably represent fragments of nuclei. Recently MURPHY et al. (1971) reported a detailed daily examination of liver-, spleen- and lung specimens of experimentally infected cercopithecans with respect to virus titers, immunofluorescence, light microscopic histology and thin section electron microscopy. Beginning with day 3 post inoculation the necrotic liver changes spread with increasing numbers of virus particles and antigen content. The most dramatic changes occurred between day 7 and 9. The liver was the primary target organ in the infection. A similar process developed in the spleen, the tissue damage did not appear, however, until somewhat later, and the virus titers did not reach the extraordinarily high level as compared with the liver. In the lung the infection remained restricted to blood vessels and macrophages.

b) Guinea Pig

The most important experimental animal is the guinea pig. Its susceptibility was discovered following inoculation with blood from the original patients. This made possible the isolation and identification of the virus (SIEGERT et al., 1967 a, b; 1968 a, c; SMITH et al., 1967; KUNZ et al., 1968 a; MAY and KNOTHE, 1968; SIMPSON et al., 1968 b; STOJKOVIĆ et al., 1971). Intraperitoneal, intravenous, intra- and subcutaneous, intracerebral, intratesticular, conjunctival, and nasal infections were all successful. The incubation period was 3–10 days long; symptoms were very few and nonspecific. As a rule, a high fever lasting 4–7 days occurred; anorexia, loss of weight, and general weakness developed, and conjunctivitis and dyspnoe were also frequently present. The animals survived the illness and were immune to reinfection (SIEGERT et al., 1967 b, 1968 a). In the course of 3–5 passages a considerable increase in virulence of the Marburg virus occurred, in which the incubation period was shortened to 1–3 days. Hihg transaminase values indicated extensive liver damage. Extreme subnormal temperatures and disturbances in blood clotting were observed before death. Even when the infectious doses were minimal, the mortality was 100 per cent. Death occurred at the latest 10–15 days after infection.

Blood and organs exhibited high concentrations of virus (10^6/ml) (SIEGERT et al., 1968 a), so that direct demonstration was possible with the electron microscope (PETERS and MÜLLER, 1968). Using the technique of immunofluorescence, viral antigen was found stored predominantly in the cytoplasm of cells of organs containing necroses. The antigen content increased considerably in the course of the passages, and was greatest in the liver, spleen, testes, peritoneal exudate, and the lungs (SLENCZKA et al., 1968). No strict correlation was found between the antigen content as determined by immunofluorescence and the extent of damage to the liver parenchymal cells (KORB and SLENCZKA, 1971). For animal experiments it should be noted that contact infections are possible among guinea pigs (SHU et al., 1968). The pathologic-anatomic changes have been studied by several teams (SMITH et al., 1967; KUNZ et al., 1968 a; BECHTELSHEIMER, 1968; SIMPSON et al., 1968 b; KORB et al., 1969; 1971; KORB and SLENCZKA, 1971; ZLOTNIK, 1969; BECHTELSHEIMER et al., 1971). The histopathologic findings were largely similar to those in patients, as well as to those in experimentally infected monkeys and hamsters. Only the interstitial pneumonitis and the hemorrhaging reported by some authors could not be confirmed by others.

Comparison of the type and development of the liver damage to that in the classic form of hepatitis in man was of particular interest. In spite of the "pantropism" of the Marburg virus, the involvement of the liver was especially conspicuous in the guinea pig, as in other subjects. Because the earliest changes in man could not be studied, BECHTELSHEIMER (1968) and BECHTELSHEIMER et al. (1971) sacrificed 20 guinea pigs between the first and the fifteenth days after infection. Acidophilic necroses of individual cells were found as early as the second and third day. These developed into disseminated focal necroses which, like those in yellow fever, underwent enlargement by concentric expansion. The hepatocyte cytoplasm contained conspicuous eosinophilic (in some cases, weakly basophilic), PAS-positive, Feulgen-negative bodies, some of which were surrounded by a lighter areola. The necrotic zones also contained round, strongly basophilic particles (1—2 μ).

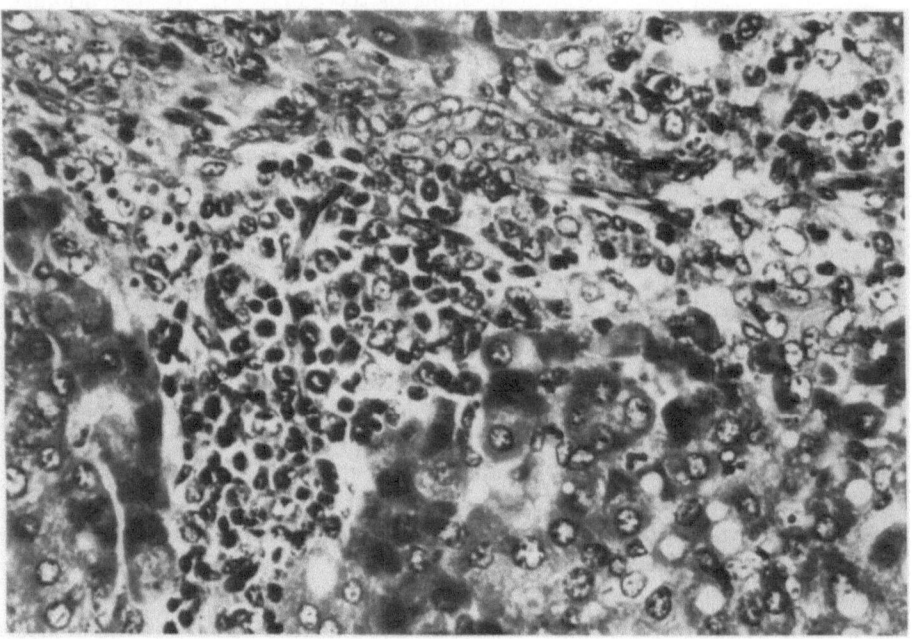

Fig. 6. Light micrograph of section of guinea pig liver ten days after infection with Marburg virus of the third passage. Portions of a periportal area with dense infiltration of monocytoid cells are visible. Formalin fixation; staining with hematoxylin-eosin (× 250). Courtesy Prof. KORB, Marburg

The development of the light microscopic changes in the liver was followed systematically by KORB and SLENCZKA (1971) and KORB et al. (1971) on a large animal collective from the first through the twenty-sixth passages (Figs. 6–10). The severity and extent of the damage increased considerably with the passage number. The hepatitis in the first passage was fully developed 8–10 days after infection, and corresponded to that observed in the patients. The symptoms underwent clear remission in the course of 2–4 weeks. Five months later, loose infiltrations of round cells in the portal areas and small nodules of stellate cells persisted in some animals as evidence of previous damage. Nevertheless, a *restitutio ad integrum* as in man can be assumed.

From the third passage onward, marked liver damage was evident as early as the third or fourth day following infection, due to the shortened incubation period.

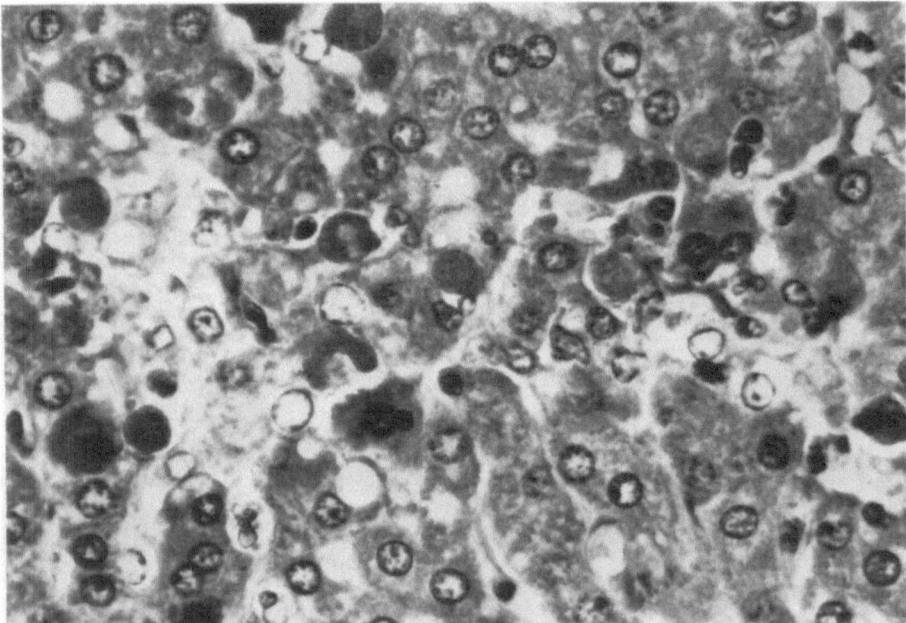

Fig. 7. Light micrograph of section of guinea pig liver, 13 days after infection with Marburg virus of the first passage. Single cell necroses of various stages are visible, some resembling so-called Councilman bodies. Formalin fixation; staining with hematoxylin-eosin (× 400). Courtesy Prof. Korb, Marburg

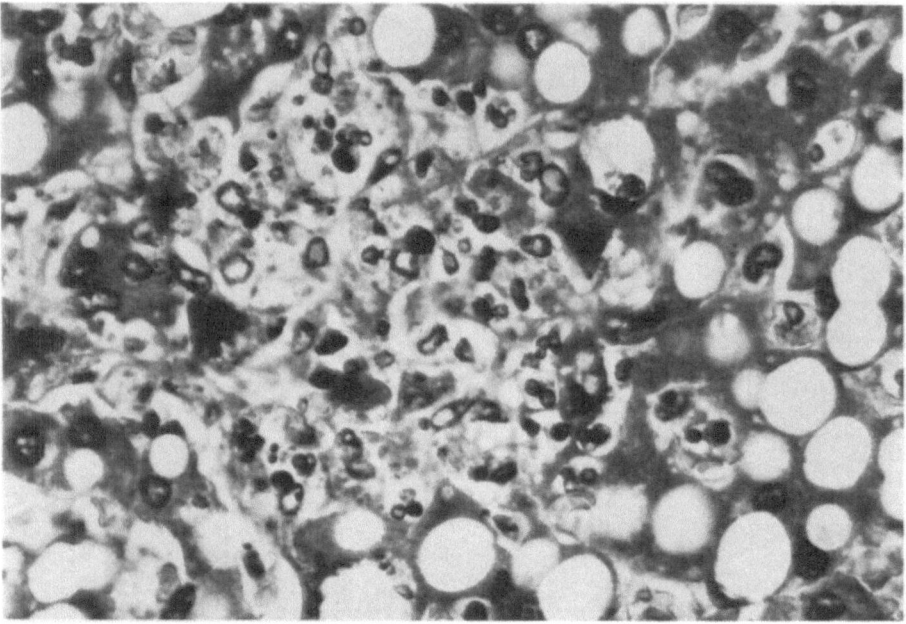

Fig. 8. Light micrograph of section of guinea pig liver, eleven days after infection with Marburg virus of the third passage. Nodule-like proliferations of stellate cells in the area of a largely absorbed focus and marked fat accumulation in the remaining hepatocytes are visible. Formalin fixation; staining with hematoxylin-eosin (× 400). Courtesy Prof. Korb, Marburg

8*

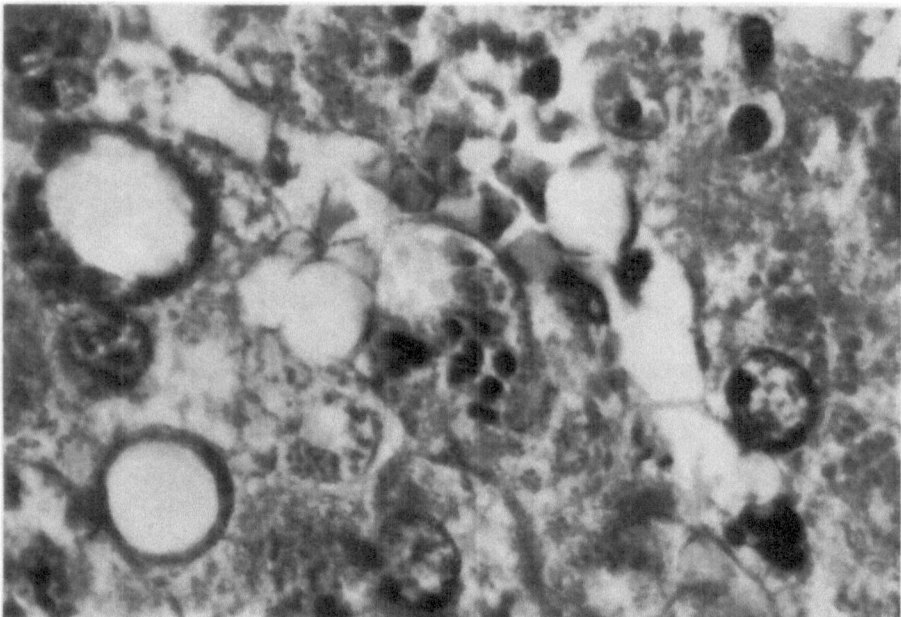

Fig. 9. Light micrograph of a section of guinea pig liver, six days after infection with Marburg virus of the 26th passage. So-called basophilic bodies and one eosinophilic inclusion with a clear halo are visible in a cell at the lower left of picture. Formalin fixation; staining with hematoxylin-eosin (× 1000). Courtesy Prof. KORB, Marburg

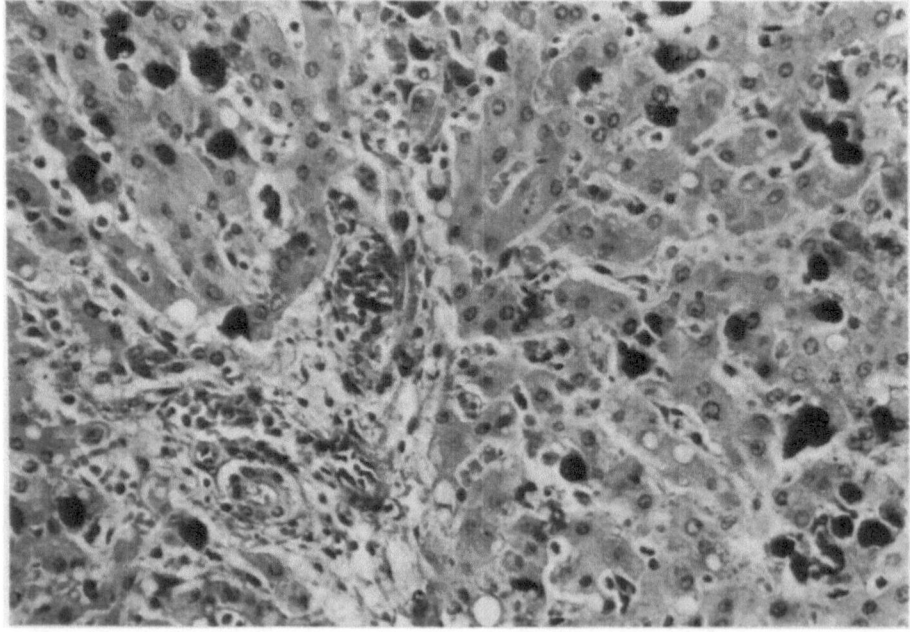

Fig. 10. Light micrograph of section of guinea pig liver, six days after infection with Marburg virus of the 23rd passage. So-called basophilic bodies, impregnated with calcium salts, are visible in the cells. Formalin fixation; von Kossa stain (× 160). Courtesy Prof. KORB, Marburg

In addition to typical coagulation necroses of the hepatocytes, "balloon cells" have been described, large numbers of which were also found in the spleen. In spite of extensive degeneration of the liver cells, Kupffer cell proliferation was present only to a minimal degree. The survival time of 6 days might have been too short for a stronger mesenchymal reaction. A special morphologic feature of hepatocytes, and occasionally of stellate cells, was the occurrence of typical, strongly basophilic structures, which increased in frequency with the passage number. These were easily distinguishable from the intra- and extracellular basophilic bodies which had been observed as early as the first passage, and consisted of extremely fine granules with a maximum diameter of 1μ. Their pathogenetic significance is still uncertain. At first they were interpreted as *rickettsiae* or members of the psittacosis-lymphogranuloma group (SMITH *et al.*, 1967; SIMPSON, 1969 c). SIMPSON *et al.* (1968 b) and ZLOTNIK (1969) suggested that these structures were the pathogen itself, surrounded by a cover supplied by the host cell and consisting of gluco- or mucopolysaccharides in which calcium salts had been precipitated. More exact information may be expected from electron microscopic and histochemical studies; only KUNZ *et al.* (1968 a) have presented data concerning the electron microscopically accessible tissue damage in the liver and spleen.

The neuropathologic changes were studied by SOLCHER (1971). Glial nodule encephalitis (Figs. 11, 12) was found in 2 out of 15 brains after intracerebral and in 3 after intraperitoneal infection, although no neurologic signs were clinically evident. The lesions affected mainly the medulla and the mesencephalon; notably

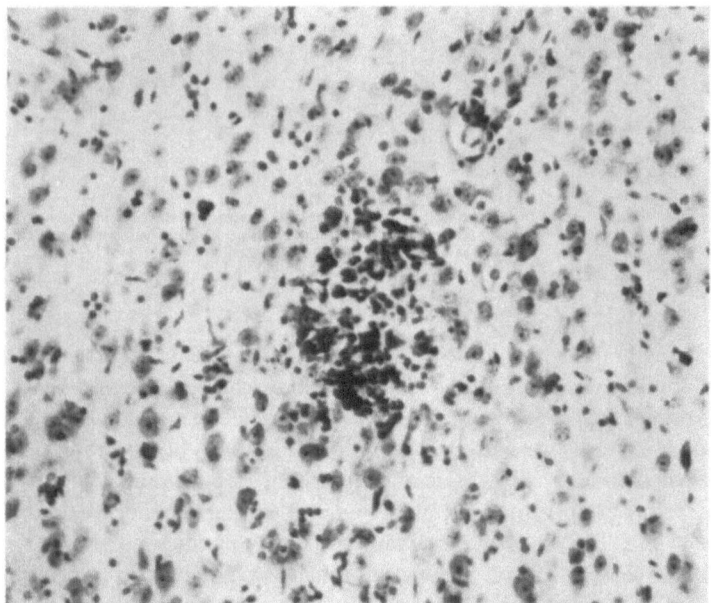

Fig. 11. Light micrograph of section of guinea pig brain after intracerebral infection with Marburg virus of the first passage. Glial nodules are visible, with particular involvement of the microglia of the brain cortex. Formalin fixation; staining with cresyl violet (× 200). Courtesy Prof. SOLCHER, Marburg

the cerebellum was not involved. In contrast, the human cases exhibited panencephalitis. The difference was attributed to species-specific variation. No relation was found between the histologic findings and the amount of antigen found by immunofluorescence.

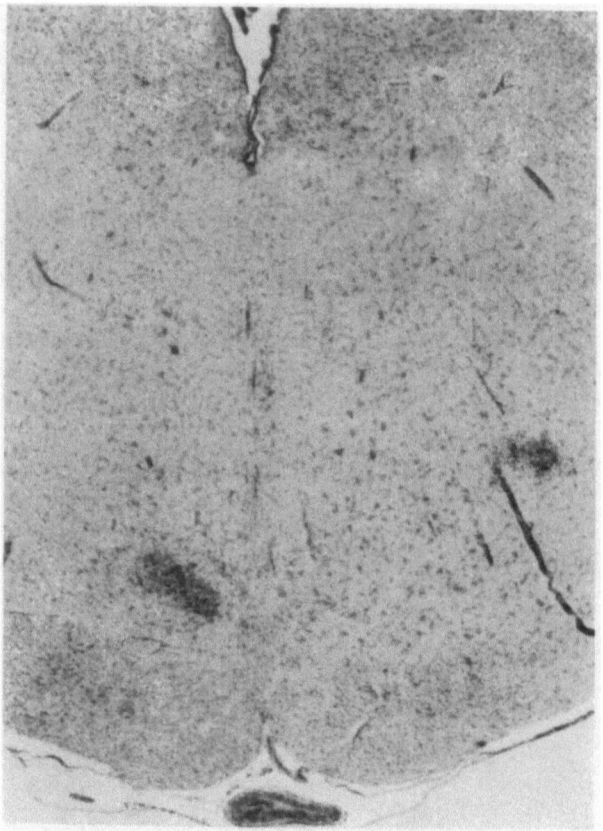

Fig. 12. Light micrograph of section of guinea pig brain stem after intraperitoneal infection with Marburg virus of the first passage. Several glial nodules are visible. Formalin fixation; staining with hematoxylin-eosin (× 28). Courtesy Prof. SOLCHER, Marburg

c) Hamsters

Adult hamsters which had received infectious material from patients in the acute stage developed no signs of illness. They did, however, become sick after inoculation with guinea pig blood from the fifth passage (SMITH et al., 1967).

The Marburg virus was successfully adapted to baby hamsters in the course of several intracerebral or intraperitoneal passages of virus-infected brain or liver tissue (SIMPSON, 1969e). In the first passage 40–80 per cent of the baby hamsters were susceptible. The mortality increased with the passage number and the incubation period became shorter. From the ninth passage onward a uniform disease developed after an incubation time of 5–9 days; it almost always ended fatally. A few animals showed signs of paralysis, indicating encephalitis. The virus appeared in particularly high concentrations in the brain. Hamsters older than

5–6 weeks developed symptoms of the illness and died only after being inoculated with material from the ninth infant hamster passage. Those animals which did not become ill or which survived the disease had antibodies and could not be reinfected.

As in the other animals, the pathologic changes in the hamster have been subjected to careful study (ZLOTNIK and SIMPSON, 1969; ZLOTNIK, 1969, 1971). Initially only slight lesions could be discerned; however, they became more severe with increasing passage numbers, until they were largely comparable to the organ damage in man, monkeys, and guinea pigs. Therefore we can dispense with a detailed description. Cerebral lesions corresponding to meningoencephalitis were a peculiar feature of the infection in hamsters; in the baby animals they were found regardless of the route of infection, but in adults they occurred only after intra-cerebral inoculation. It should nevertheless be mentioned that similar changes in the brain have also been reported in experimentally infected guinea pigs (SOLCHER, 1971).

In the brain the process consisted of microglial and astroglial proliferation, hemorrhages, and neuronal degeneration. Perivascular lymphocytic cuffings were not present. After 5 passages changes were also present in the kidneys and lungs. It was regarded as especially interesting that the basophilic cytoplasmic inclusions after 9 passages appeared not only in the liver, as in the guinea pig, but in cells of the kidneys and lungs as well. They were Feulgen- and PAS-positive, and were interpreted as being accumulations of the pathogenic agent (SIMPSON et al., 1968 b; ZLOTNIK, 1969). A definitive answer depends on further histochemical, fluorescence-serologic, and electron microscopic studies.

d) Mice

Adult mice developed no pathologic symptoms following inoculation with patients' blood or passage material from guinea pigs (SMITH et al., 1967; MAY and KNOTHE, 1968). Even after repeated passages through mice, no evidence could be found indicating replication of the virus. Nevertheless, it proved possible to adapt the agent to the brains of baby mice by means of several intracerebral passages, without development of symptoms (KUNZ et al., 1968 a). Even after 20 passages the infection produced no symptoms. The mouse-adapted virus retained its pathogenicity for guinea pigs and produced a cytopathic effect in ELF (embryonic human lung fibroblasts) cells (HOFMANN and KUNZ, 1971). In 57 mice which had been inoculated intracerebrally or intraperitoneally, in some cases combined with subcutaneous injections, at ages of up to 48 hours and which had been examined 3–40 days later, no symptoms and no histologic lesions could be found; the only exception was a single mouse whose brain cells contained eosinophilic inclusion bodies (MALHERBE and STRICKLAND-CHOLMLEY, 1971). No inclusions of antigenic material were present in adult mice 7 and 14 days after intracerebral or intraperitoneal infection. The blood from several mice was pooled 6 weeks after infection; it had a complement-fixing antibody titer of 1 : 32 with cell culture antigens (SLENCZKA and WOLFF, 1971). The mute course of the infection in mice hardly seems traceable to interferon, for the latter could not be demonstrated in mouse brains (HOFMANN and KUNZ, 1969 b).

A virus strain which initially had an infectious, but not pathogenic potential for baby mice acquired a pathogenicity for these animals during three passages in hamsters, and was thereby capable of inducing fatal encephalitis (HOFMANN and KUNZ, 1970). In the course of further baby mouse passages the virulence increased, as well as the concentration of the virus in the brain ($10^{3.2}$ LD$_{50}$ in the 3rd passage, $10^{5.5}$ LD$_{50}$ in the 8th passage). The antigen could be demonstrated by immunofluorescence, and showed positive reactions with antisera in the complement fixation test. Adult mice were also resistant to the neuro-adapted virus strain.

e) Other Hosts

Intrathoracic multiplication of the Marburg virus was possible in *Aedes aegypti*, but not in *Anopheles maculipennis* or *Ixodes ricinus* (KUNZ et al., 1968 b; HOFMANN et al., 1969; KUNZ and HOFMANN, 1971). Although it would be of great epidemiologic and taxonomic interest to know whether the virus can be transmitted by *Aedes*, this problem has not yet been studied, due to the risk inherent in such experiments.

Multiplication of the agent in the chick embryo was not observed following either inoculation of the yolk sac or of the chorioallantoic membrane (SMITH et al., 1967; MAY and KNOTHE, 1968).

2. Virus Multiplication

The replication of the Marburg virus is understood only in its rough features, for studies at the molecular level in particular are still lacking. The first clues concerning the replication were reported by SIEGERT et al. (1967 a, b). The viral antigen has been found only in the cytoplasm and (in rare cases) extracellularly, but never in the nucleus of the host cell. The largest inclusions were observed at the cell membrane, which they appeared to cause to bulge outward. The occurrence of finger-like protrusions and bud-like processes on the surface of the cell suggests that extrusion proceeds by budding.

Electron microscopic evidence, too, indicates that morphogenesis occurs only in the cytoplasm and in association with the process of extrusion, without apparent involvement of the nucleus (Figs. 13–19). HÜLSER (1969) has studied the development within human amniotic cells and found the agent in small colonies within the cytoplasm. The envelope was still lacking and was formed in the course of extrusion. Enveloped virus particles were found almost exclusively outside the cell.

ALMEIDA et al. (1971) have drawn conclusions concerning the morphogenesis from the ultrastructure as revealed in negative staining. They consider the naked helix with its central core to be the primary component of the virus. The existence of intermediate forms suggests that it receives an investing membrane, thereby becoming the internal component of the coiled and circular (torus) forms. The inner helix is remarkably similar to that of other viruses, e. g., the measles virus (WATERSON, 1965). The structure is completed by a superficial membrane which probably contains lipid and exhibits projections on its surface. Maturation of the virus seems to occur with the bending of the "full", coiled particles to circular structures, which are found in large aggregations.

The successive stages of development have been studied systematically by PETERS et al. (1971) on sections of infected Vero cells (Figs. 13–19). After 8 hours neither viral particles of the inoculum nor signs of a new virus generation could be found. The first changes were observed 24 hours after infection and consisted of accumulations of blurred, wavy filaments (diameter about 55 mμ) in the

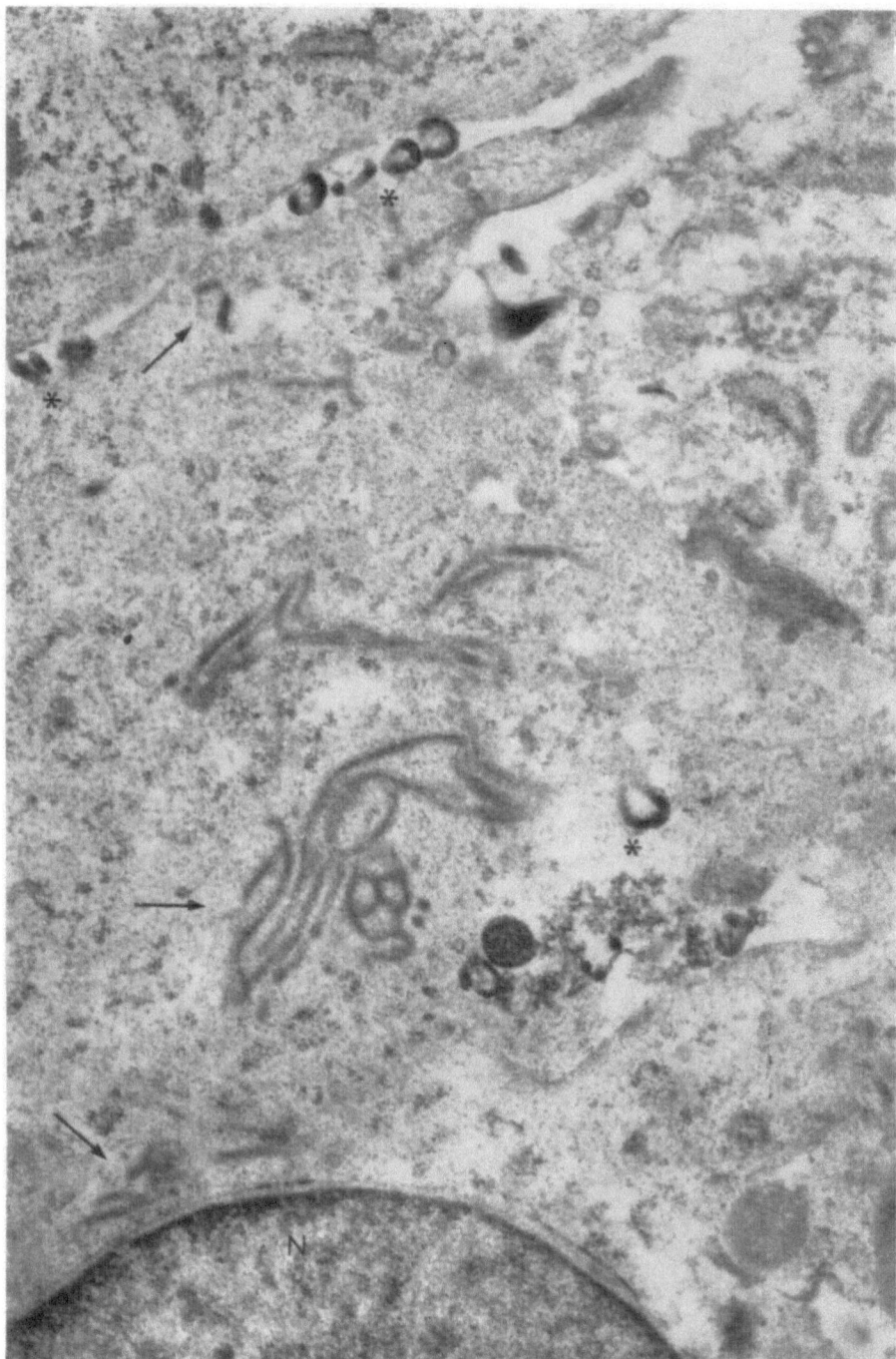

Fig. 13. Electron micrograph of an infected Vero cell 32 hours after infection, showing virus particles without envelopes in the cytoplasm (arrows), more strongly contrasted virus particles with envelopes within a cytoplasmic vesicle and an intercellular space (asterisks), and the nucleus (N). Glutar- and formaldehyde fixation; embedding in Epon; staining with UO₂-acetate and Pb-citrate (× 20,000). Courtesy Prof. PETERS and Dr. MÜLLER, Hamburg

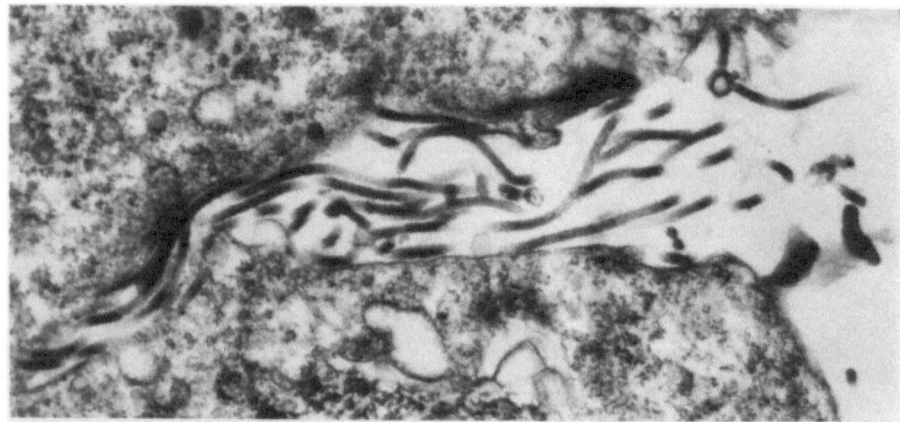

Fig. 14. Electron micrograph of infected Vero cells 48 hours after infection, showing straight, intercellular virus particles. Preparation as in Fig. 13 (× 17,000). Courtesy Prof PETERS and Dr. MÜLLER, Hamburg

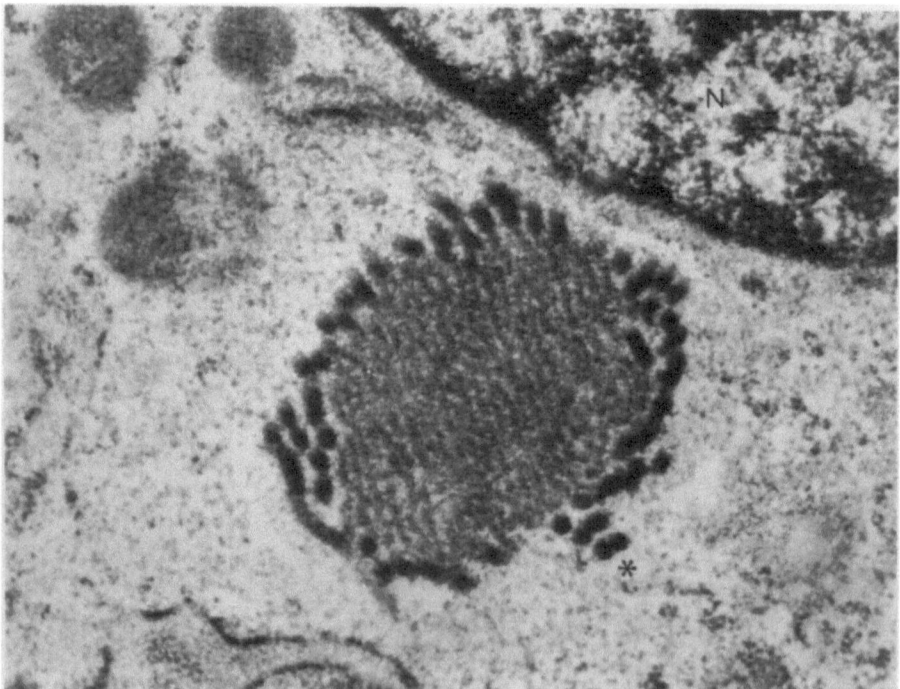

Fig. 15. Electron micrograph of an intracytoplasmic inclusion body in a Vero cell three days after infection. Fine filaments are visible in the center and denser strands in the periphery, some of which show electron lucent cores (asterisk). Nucleus (N). Preparation as in Fig. 13 (× 35,000). Courtesy Prof. PETERS and Dr. MÜLLER, Hamburg

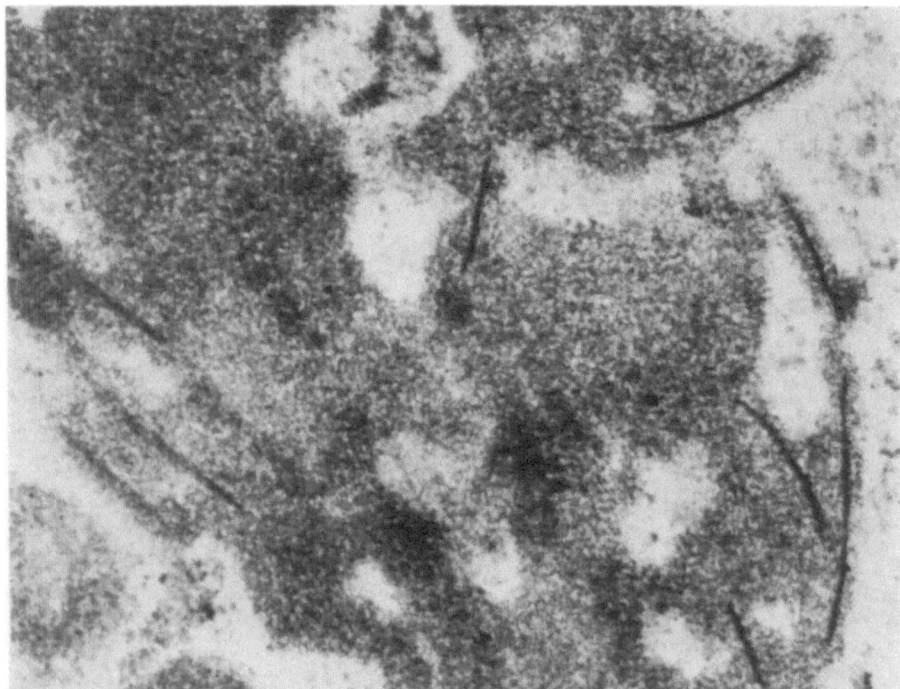

Fig. 16. Electron micrograph of an intracytoplasmic inclusion body in a Vero cell five days after infection, showing electron opaque lamellae embedded in matrix. Preparation as in Fig. 13 (× 40,000). Courtesy Prof. PETERS and Dr. MÜLLER, Hamburg

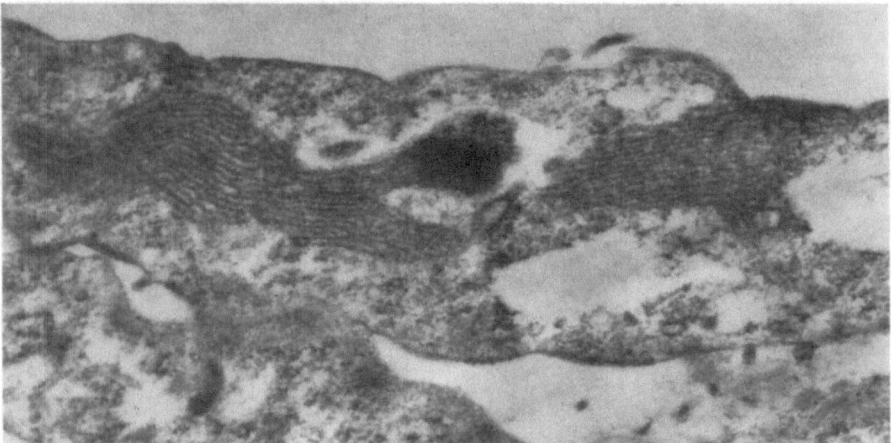

Fig. 17. Electron micrograph of intracytoplasmic inclusion bodies in a Vero cell three days after infection. The inclusion bodies consist of aggregations of naked nucleocapsids. Preparation as in Fig. 13 (× 20,000). Courtesy Prof. PETERS and Dr. MÜLLER, Hamburg

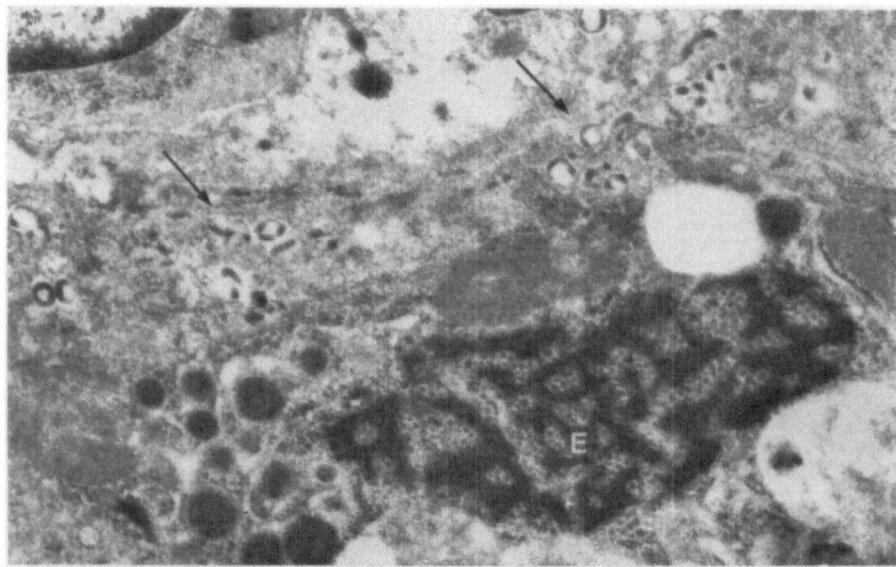

Fig. 18. Electron micrograph of an intracytoplasmic inclusion body (E) in an infected guinea pig liver cell. Virus particles are visible in vesicles (arrows) in the periphery of the cell. Preparation as in Fig. 13 (× 15,000). Courtesy Prof. PETERS and Dr. MÜLLER, Hamburg

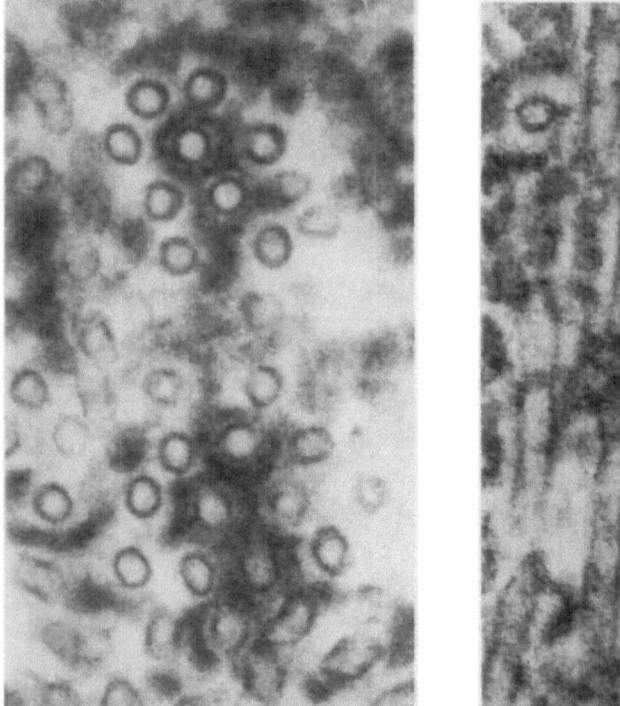
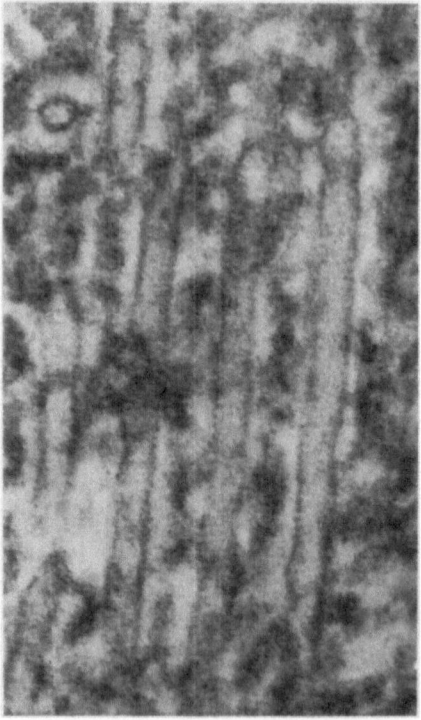

Fig. 19. Electron micrograph of an intracytoplasmic inclusion body of the type shown in Fig. 17, five days after infection. Loosely arranged nucleocapsids with portions of matrix. a) Transverse section of the same inclusion body, showing hexagonal arrangement (× 200,000). b) Longitudinal section of the inclusion body, showing 53 Å cross striations (× 200,000). Preparation as in Fig. 13. Courtesy Prof. PETERS and Dr. MÜLLER, Hamburg

cytoplasm. It is possible that they represent ultrastructural equivalents of the virus-specific inclusions which can be made visible at this stage with immuno-fluorescence. After 32 hours more widely scattered, straight strands were seen. Complete virus entities (straight, coiled, and ring-shaped particles) had budded from the cell membrane into cytoplasmic vesicles and into the extracellular spaces. Budding itself was seen only rarely. The cytoplasmic virus strands probably represent the nucleocapsid and intermediate layer. According to these studies, the envelope is added only during extrusion. The typical pleomorphism indicates great flexibility of the inner strand; the manner by which the straight rods bend to form coils or rings is not yet clear. This transformation process always involves only one end of the rod (MAY and HERZBERG, 1969).

As a further electron microscopic manifestation of the cellular infection, PETERS et al. (1971) described compact cytoplasmic inclusion bodies of notable variability (Figs. 15–19). The first appeared in Vero cells and in experimental animals 32 hours following infection, and are identical with the Negri-type inclusions seen in light microscopy (PETERS and MÜLLER, 1969 b). The observation that different kinds of inclusions occur in different types of cells seems to possess general validity (PETERS, 1969). For instance, spongy-looking aggregations of strands were often observed. Characteristic of another type is a concentric arrangement of the strands to form lamellar or palisade-like subunits. Other inclusions exhibit a center filled with delicate filaments, whereas the periphery contains heavily stained strands. The latter and a yet further type, in which lamellae and spheres occur in bizarre arrangements embedded in a matrix, are reminiscent of inclusions found in cells infected with rabies (HUMMELER et al., 1967). Other types resemble inclusions of vesicular stomatitis (DAVID-WEST and LABZOFFSKY, 1968) or of Egtved virus (ZWILLENBERG et al., 1965). Both of these are arranged in a regular, hexagonal pattern of closely-packed nucleocapsids. The beadstring-like structure of the nucleocapsid helix is revealed in suitably oriented cross sections.

Presumably the compact cellular inclusions do not represent any particular stage in the development of the virus. PETERS et al. (1971) consider them to be abortive structures consisting of surplus virus-specific material. Possibly they are derived from the loose aggregations of strands found in the early stages of replication of the virus.

Recently MURPHY et al. (1971) followed the kinetics of viral maturation in liver cells of experimentally infected cercopithecans by negative contrast technique. They found important differences in the morphogenesis between the Marburg virus and the rhabdoviruses which not only concerned the cross-sectional character of the mature virus particles but also the nature of the cellular inclusions. Rhabdoviruses consist of a double ring, but the proportion of central space is very large relative to that in Marburg virus. This difference in central core size is fundamental. The Rhabdovirus inclusion, e.g. the matrix in rabies virus-infected cells consists of massed, unorganized ribonucleoprotein strands. In contrast, Marburg virus inclusion bodies become extremely structured.

3. Cytopathogenicity

The Marburg virus is capable of replication in cell cultures of various origin, and often reaches high titers in the cultural supernatants; nevertheless, a consider-

able amount of virus usually retains its association with the cell. Cytopathic
effects were observed only in a few primary and permanent cell culture systems
(Tables 1 and 2). The discrepancies in the data of various authors are presumably
due mostly to differing experimental conditions or procedures.

Table 1. *Propagation of Marburg Virus in Primary Cell Cultures*
(supplemented after HOFMANN and KUNZ, 1971)

Primary cells	Virus replication	CPE	Virus titer	References
Cercopithecus kidney	+	—	n. d.[a]	SIEGERT et al. (1968 b)
Cercopithecus kidney	+	—	n. d.	MALHERBE and STRICKLAND-CHOLMLEY (1968, 1971)
Cercopithecus kidney	+	+	n. d.	HAAS et al. (1968 b)
Rhesus kidney	+	—	n. d.	HOFMANN and KUNZ (1968)
Human amnion	+	+/—	n. d.	MAY et al. (1968)
Human amnion	—			MALHERBE and STRICKLAND-CHOLMLEY (1971)
Human leukocytes		—		MAY and KNOTHE (1968)
Chick embryo fibroblasts	+	—	10^1 [b]	HOFMANN and KUNZ (1968)
Chick embryo fibroblasts	—			SMITH et al. (1967)
Chick embryo fibroblasts		—	n. d.	MAY and KNOTHE (1968)
Guinea pig fibroblasts	+	—	10^3 [b]	HOFMANN and KUNZ (1968)
Guinea pig kidney		—	n. d.	MAY and KNOTHE (1968)

[a]) not determined
[b]) assayed in guinea pigs

The first report of a cytopathic effect (CPE) of the Marburg virus came from
ZLOTNIK et al. (1968 a). On the fifth day after infection of BHK-21 cell cultures
they found that 20 per cent of the cells contained inclusion bodies. An incomplete
cytopathic effect developed by the thirteenth day. In the third and fourth passages
the inclusions were already present on the first day, and cytopathic changes could
be seen by the seventh. HOFMANN and KUNZ (1968) found a weak CPE somewhat
later, whereas KISSLING et al. (1968) observed its appearance as early as between
the second and fifth days in a highly susceptible cell strain. Virus titrations were
difficult, for the control cultures which had not been inoculated remained in good
condition for only 7–8 days. The virus titer increased within a few culture
passages from 10^{-3} to $10^{-6.5}$ TCID$_{50}$/0.1 ml. In contrast to SIEGERT et al. (1968 b)
and MALHERBE and STRICKLAND-CHOLMLEY (1968), HAAS et al. (1968 b) found a
marked CPE in primary cultures of Cercopithecus kidney cells; the effect increased
considerably in the course of 5 passages. The virus concentration reached a

Table 2. *Propagation of Marburg Virus in Established Cell Lines*
(supplemented after Hofmann and Kunz, 1971)

Cell line	Virus replication	CPE	Virus titer	References
Cercopithecus kidney (CMK-AH$_1$)	+	−	10^6 [a]	Hofmann and Kunz (1968)
Cercopithecus kidney (CMK-AH$_1$)	+	+ (2–5)[b]	n. d.[c]	Kissling et al. (1968)
Vero	+	−	n. d.	Siegert et al. (1968 b)
Vero	+	+/−	n. d.	Kissling et al. (1968)
Vero	+	+(3–10)[b]	n. d.	Slenczka (1969 a, b)
Vero	+	−	n. d.	Malherbe and Strickland-Cholmley (1971)
Cynomolgus heart (CMH)	+	−	10^1 [a]	Hofmann and Kunz (1968)
Rhesus kidney (LLC-MK$_2$)	−		n. d.	Smith et al. (1967)
Rhesus kidney (LLC-MK$_2$)	+	−	n. d.	Malherbe and Strickland-Cholmley (1971)
L (mouse embryo)	−			Hofmann and Kunz (1968)
L (mouse embryo)	+	−	n. d.	Smith et al. (1967)
Guinea pig heart	+	−	n. d.	Kissling et al. (1968)
BHK-21	+	+/−	10^1 [a]	Hofmann and Kunz (1968)
BHK-21	+	+ (7–23)[b]	n. d.	Zlotnik et al. (1968 a)
BHK-21 (W 12)	+	+/−	n. d.	Kissling et al. (1968)
BHK-21 (CCL 10)	+	+ (2–5)[b]	$10^{6.5}$ [d]	Kissling et al. (1968)
BHK-21	+	−	n. d.	Malherbe and Strickland-Cholmley (1971)
HeLa	+	−	10^4 [a]	Hofmann and Kunz (1968)
HeLa	−		n. d.	Siegert et al. (1968 b)
HeLa	−		n. d.	Smith et al. (1967)
HeLa	−	−	n. d.	May and Knothe (1968)
HeLa	+	−	n. d.	Malherbe and Strickland-Cholmley (1971)
WI 38	+	−	n. d.	Malherbe and Strickland-Cholmley (1971)
Foreskin fibroblasts	+	+[e]	n. d.	Kissling et al. (1968)
U (human amnion)	+	−	n. d.	Hofmann and Kunz (1971)
ELF (embryonic human lung fibroblasts)	+	+ (3–5)[b]	10^6 [a] 10^4 [d]	Hofmann and Kunz (1970)

[a] assayed in guinea pigs   [b] in brackets: days   [c] not determined
[d] assayed in tissue culture   [e] not in serial passages

maximum of $10^{7.3}$ TCID$_{50}$/ml. However, the monkey cells in culture proved to be less susceptible than subcutaneously infected cercopithecans. Neither alteration of the incubation temperature nor addition of cortisone (20 µg/ml) to the medium could stimulate replication of the Marburg virus (MALHERBE and STRICKLAND-CHOLMLEY, 1971). In a permanent cell line derived from Cercopithecus kidney a total CPE on the fourth to fifth day was described by KISSLING et al. (1968), whereas HOFMANN and KUNZ (1968) were not able to find any, in spite of highly active virus replication. MAY and HERZBERG (1969) succeeded in adapting a strain which had been cultivated in guinea pigs to human amnion cells. The CPE was fully developed by the fifth day; the titers in this culture were $10^{-6.5}$ to 10^{-7}. HOFMANN and KUNZ (1971) reported a definite but incomplete CPE in ELF cells (embryonic human lung fibroblasts); a maximum was attained on the fifth day. The CPE began in spindle-shaped foci and later involved clumping of the cells. The virus titer reached 10^{-4} to 10^{-6}, as determined by the infection of guinea pigs, which proved to be more susceptible than ELF cells.

Since the CPE was usually lacking, the appearance of cytoplasmic inclusions became an important indicator for the degree of virus multiplication in cell cultures. Direct and indirect immunofluorescence according to COONS has proved especially suitable for demonstration of the presence of virus (SIEGERT et al., 1967 b; 1968 b; SLENCZKA et al., 1968; CARTER and BRIGHT, 1968; SLENCZKA, 1969 a, b; MAASS et al., 1969). Inclusion bodies are also visible in phase-contrast microscopy (SIEGERT et al., 1968 b) and can be stained using various methods. In preparations stained with hematoxylin-eosin, eosinophilic, Feulgen-negative inclusions have been observed (MALHERBE and STRICKLAND-CHOLMLEY, 1968; 1971; MAASS et al., 1969). Sellers' stain (methylene blue — fuchsin), which is used for demonstration of Negri bodies, was shown to be just as useful as immunofluorescence (SLENCZKA, 1969 a, b). There was a direct proportionality between the virus concentration and the number of infected cells.

Following large doses of virus, inclusions were apparent as early as the third to fifth day in BHK and Vero cells (Figs. 5 a–c) and in primary cultures of simian kidney fibroblasts. With increasing numbers of passages and duration of the incubation period they grew considerably in size (from 5 µ initially to 10 µ and more) and in number, so that finally almost all cells were filled with antigen. The latent period between infection and development of the inclusions was reduced in the course of three passages to 24 hours. After several passages a cytopathic effect developed with high infectious doses. In Vero cells this CPE could be inhibited by addition of human or bovine serum. No plaque formation occurred under an overlay of 0.5 per cent agarose (SLENCZKA, 1969 a, b).

SLENCZKA and WOLFF (1971) succeeded in infecting a Vero cell line "chronically" with Marburg virus adapted to the host cell in the course of 6 passages. Subcultures of the last passage were made on the fourth day. Although the viral antigen was found in more than 90 per cent of the cells, no CPE developed. The rate of growth of the carrier cells did not differ from that of the normal control cultures. In the fifth subculture the virus concentration was 10^5 to 10^6 ID$_{50}$/ml. The mechanism of the carrier state in which no antiserum is necessary is not fully understood. It is not known whether interferon is involved. Vero carrier cells were used as a source of a complement-fixing antigen (p. 108).

As studies on primary kidney cell cultures from experimentally infected vervet monkeys have shown, the infection with Marburg virus does not interfere with cell proliferation. Subculturing was also possible. No cytopathic effect was observed. On the second day following inoculation, however, varying numbers of cells of the culture were found to contain eosinophilic inclusions in the cytoplasm, visible under high-power magnification. The virus-specific antigen could be detected by immunofluorescence. In addition, numerous viral particles were demonstrated electron microscopically (MAASS et al., 1969; HAAS and MAASS, 1971). The Marburg virus survived trypsin treatment as used in the preparation of cell cultures (BOWEN et al., 1969; MAASS et al., 1969). The virus also multiplied in poliovirus infected primary monkey cell cultures, where it is likewise recognizable on the basis of the characteristic inclusions (MALHERBE and STRICKLAND-CHOLMLEY, 1971).

With regard to the production of vaccines in primary monkey kidney cells, it was of great practical interest to know whether the presence of Marburg virus would affect the multiplication of poliovirus. MALHERBE and STRICKLAND-CHOLMLEY (1971) found the development of the CPE of poliovirus to be delayed by 24 hours. They observed eosinophilic, cytoplasmic inclusions of Marburg virus in cell cultures simultaneously infected with poliovirus. Cells infected with both foamy agent and Marburg virus formed syncytia with thread-like inclusions in the cytoplasm. When the occurrence of both cell reactions is encountered, the possibility of a double infection should be borne in mind. The same authors note that parainfluenza type 1 also induces syncytia formation with inclusions, but this is followed by complete destruction of the cell layer.

F. Pathogenesis

Experimental infections of monkeys always proved fatal, even when extremely small amounts of the pathogen were involved. It did not matter whether transmission was made by injection, by direct contact, or indirectly. Whereas lethality was 100 per cent in cercopithecans and macaques, 22 per cent of the human patients died, while hamsters and guinea pigs survived the first passage without losses. In the course of further homologous passages a considerable enhancement in virulence occurred with increasing adaptation. In retransfer of infectious blood from patients or guinea pigs to monkeys, the original high virulence was found to be undiminished. This documents the difference in pathogenicity of the Marburg virus for various hosts.

1. In Humans

The virus-host relationships are shown in Table 3. According to STILLE et al. (1968), the manifestation of this infectious disease involves 3 phases: Viremia is followed by early organ involvement (skin rash, hepatitis, leukocytosis, hemorrhagic diatheses, etc.). Occasionally a late organ phase was also observed (myocarditis, orchitis, edema, symptoms of encephalitis). In the opinion of STILLE and BÖHLE (1971), the persistence of virocytes in follow-up examinations is indicative of a chronic, latent infection.

Table 3. *Virus-Host Relationships between Marburg Virus and Man*

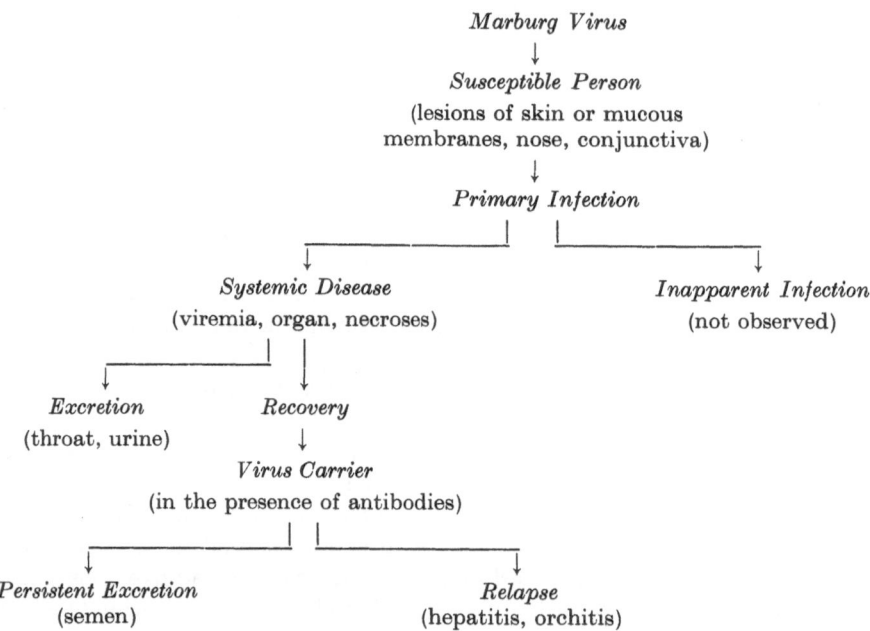

The sites of entry of the agent were lesions of the skin and mucous membranes (p. 142). In primary infections the period of incubation was 3–7 days, and in human secundary cases 5–9 days. These differences may be attributed to different infectious doses, as well as to varying degrees of virulence of the pathogen.

The viremic phase was characterized by high fever. It lasted 14 days on the average, during which virus concentrations of up to 10^4 infectious units for guinea pigs/ml plasma were reached. The agent is pantropic, and caused necroses in nearly all organs (p. 137). In some patients with enanthema and renal involvement its excretion was demonstrated in throat washing and in the urine.

All seven deaths occurred in patients who had contracted the disease directly from monkeys or from simian cell cultures. In contrast, those cases which arose after passage of the virus through humans were less severe and not fatal. This suggests an attenuation of virulence; it could also be a result of lower infectious doses.

Of special pathologic interest was the discovery that two patients continued to harbor the virus, in spite of the presence of circulating antibodies in their blood. One latent and persistent infection could be demonstrated in the semen of a excretor, who infected his wife about 11 weeks after his own recovery (MARTINI and SCHMIDT, 1968; SIEGERT et al., 1968 b, c). However, three additional convalescent patients examined in this regard were found to be negative. Persistence of virus in the semen could be followed for only about eight weeks, for impotence then occurred. In addition, Marburg virus was demonstrated in liver biopsy material taken during a relapse of hepatitis around 80 days after onset of the disease, but the blood was free of virus. The presence of neutralizing antibody prevented hematogenous spread of the pathogen, confining the relapse to the affected organ (SIEGERT *et al.*, 1968 b, c). No further evidence is available concerning the frequency of virus persistence, its duration, or its consequences. The prognosis, based on results of repeated follow-up examinations of all patients, appears nevertheless to be good (MARTINI, 1971; STILLE and BÖHLE, 1971).

The possible existence of clinically inapparent infections was also a question of significance. For this reason SLENCZKA *et al.* (1970) carried out serologic studies on 51 persons who had been exposed to the disease in much the same way as the patients. The serum samples were taken concurrently with the outbreak, and then a few months thereafter. The lack of complement-fixing antibody in this group of contact persons makes inapparent infections appear unlikely.

Finally, it is worth mentioning that three patients gave birth to healthy children 20–23 months after having been ill with the Marburg virus disease. It was not possible to demonstrate either antigen or virus in two of the placentas or in the serum of the mothers or of the babies. The passive immunity of the infants disappeared after about three months (SLENCZKA, 1970).

Animal experiments were performed in order to cast light on certain special problems of pathogenesis. The observation of excretion of the virus with the semen raised the question of the possibility of transfer of the virus to the progeny, especially since testes and ovaries of many patients were particularly affected. Because of its basic biologic-epidemiologic importance this problem was pursued by SLENCZKA and WOLFF (1971) using a guinea pig model.

No evidence was found for vertical transmission. In two pregnant animals which had been infected near the end of the period of gestation, infectious virus and cytoplasmic inclusions were found in maternal organs only, but not in placental or fetal tissue. This does not, however, refute the possibility of a germinal transmission.

A further pathogenetic problem of significance concerns the persistence of the virus. SLENCZKA and WOLFF (1971) infected newborn mice intracerebrally within the first 24 hours with material from the first to third mouse passages. In the first fourteen days they found specific antigenic inclusions predominantly in brain cells, but also in liver and spleen. After six weeks the blood was no longer infectious for guinea pigs, and showed complement-fixing antibody titers ranging from 1 : 8 to 1 : 32. Despite the presence of antibody, antigenic inclusions were still found in two mice. About 30 per cent of the neonatally infected mice which survived the first four weeks were retarded in their development and appeared sickly.

In the organs of the sick animals the number of cells containing inclusions was clearly greater than that in mice without symptoms of the illness. Surprisingly, histopathologic alterations were absent in liver, spleen, and brains of the mice which died, so that it may be questioned whether the Marburg virus was the cause of their deaths. A fully satisfactory answer concerning persistence and vertical transmission of the pathogen would require studies on the second generation of mice.

The possibility of involvement of immune processes in the development of the tissue lesions (HAAS *et al.*, 1968 a) was reexamined by KORB and SLENCZKA (1971), who treated guinea pigs with cyclophosphamide (Endoxan®) daily (10 mg/kg) for four to six days prior to infection. The damage to the liver seems to have been influenced in that hardly any mesenchymal reaction occurred. Since utilization coagulopathy appeared in the guinea pigs as well as in the patients (EGBRING *et al.*, 1971), the animals were given 250 I. U. heparin/kg daily for four to six days before infection. No influence of the heparin was apparent, however.

The single-cell and focal necroses in the liver are probably a direct deleterious effect of the Marburg virus, for the presence of agent and antigen in liver cells has been demonstrated by means of both electron microscopy and fluorescence serology. Monocytic and lymphocytic infiltration of the portal areas was interpreted as an immune response to the pathogen, and the focal necroses as a consequence of circulatory disturbances within the liver (KORB and SLENCZKA, 1971).

Regarding the hemorrhagic diathesis in the Marburg virus disease, EGBRING *et al.* (1971) analyzed the coagulation process in infected guinea pigs to see whether the thrombopenia is accompanied by any deficiencies involving plasmatic clotting factors. They were able to show that a reduction of various clotting factors of the plasma (II, V, VII, VIII, and X) occurred in the course of the disease. Corresponding to these findings, the recalcification and thromboplastin times were abnormal; the levels of the other factors were within the normal range. The severe coagulopathy and thrombopenia were interpreted as resulting from disseminated intravascular coagulation, indicated by clots of platelets and fibrin. Guinea pig blood taken in terminal stages clotted only after addition of calcium.

2. In Experimental Animals

The pathogenesis of the Marburg virus infection in animals corresponds largely to that observed in man. In experimentally infected monkeys the mean incubation period was three to four days, whereas in cases acquired by contact with animals in neighboring cages it was six to nine days. Viremia could be demonstrated even before the rise in body temperature. Unusually high concentrations of virus in the blood (10^{10}/ml) were determined in the very sensitive monkey test (HAAS *et al.*, 1968 b; SIMPSON, 1969 d). As in man, excretion of the pathogen occurs; virus concentrations of up to 10^6/ml have been found in the urine (SIMPSON *et al.*, 1968 a; SIMPSON, 1969 d). Another factor assumed to be of significance in the pathogenetic mechanism was the almost complete failure of the reticuloendothelial system, due to destruction of the reticular cells in the spleen and lymph nodes, as well as of Kupffer's stellate cells in the liver. The intravascular fibrin and platelet clots were interpreted as part of a generalized Shwartzman-Sanarelli phenomenon, and the bleeding tendency as utilization coagulopathy. No information is available about persistent infections in monkeys. A very detailed pathogenic study was recently published by MURPHY *et al.* (1971). They followed the kinetics of virus multiplication and the development of the histologic reactions in liver, spleen and lung. The tissue damage became apparent by day 3 and reached the climax in correspondance with the virus concentration between day 7 and 9.

Guinea pigs and hamsters also show generalized virus infection with involvement of all organs. The blood contained 10^6 infectious units/ml for guinea pigs (SIEGERT *et al.*, 1968 a, b; MAY and KNOTHE, 1968). The occurrence of contact infections suggests that the virus is excreted (SHU *et al.*, 1968); still, this has not been confirmed by isolation of the agent. In one guinea pig virus antigen was found in the spleen twelve days after return of the temperature to normal, but the blood was free of it. Relapses must be reckoned with in guinea pigs as in humans (MAY and KNOTHE, 1968), but a febrile reaction without isolation of the virus is no proof of a relapse.

G. Immunity

Infection with Marburg virus induces a strong immunity. Convalescent guinea pigs remained afebrile after reinfection with the same amount of virus (SIEGERT et al., 1967 b; 1968 a). The immune animals were in possession of neutralizing and complement-fixing antibodies in serum dilutions of up to 1 : 320 (p. 107, 108).

The patients likewise developed neutralizing as well as complement-fixing antibodies. Maximum titers were reached in three to four weeks and, with a single exception, antibody could still be demonstrated 14 to 20 months later (p. 141). The duration of the immunity is still unknown.

Two infants born to mothers who had been ill with the disease 20 and 23 months previously, respectively, were shown to contain transplacentally transmitted complement-fixing antibodies at birth. The passive immunity disappeared in the course of three months (SLENCZKA, 1970).

IV. Clinico-Pathologic Features

A. Clinical Symptoms

The 31 patients included 11 women; those who fell ill were all adults between 19 and 64 years of age. After the initial experience the principal symptoms were so characteristic that the clinical diagnosis could be made with great certainty, in spite of differences in degree of severity. Detailed descriptions of the clinical picture have been published by MARTINI et al., 1968 a, b; MARTINI and SCHMIDT, 1968; STILLE et al., 1968; MARTINI, 1969; MARTINI and SIEGERT, 1971; MARTINI, 1971; STILLE and BÖHLE, 1971; and TODOROVITCH et al., 1971.

The disease, which is characterized as an exanthematous, hemorrhagic fever, has entered the literature under various names. In the vernacular it was initially referred to as the "Marburger Affenkrankheit" (MARTINI et al., 1968 b; GEDIGK et al., 1968), because by far the most cases occurred in Marburg. After discovery and naming of the pathogenic agent, the syndrome was designated as the "Marburg virus disease". The names "green monkey disease" and "vervet monkey disease" (STILLE et al., 1968; SIMPSON et al., 1968 a) have also been used. Finally, it has also been referred to as the "Frankfurt-Marburg syndrome" (HAAS et al., 1968 b).

After an incubation period of from three to nine days (mean: five days), the prodromal stage set in, which was usually short. The illness began suddenly with extreme malaise, pains in the limbs, and frontal and temporal headache. Within a few hours the fever increased to 39° C without rigors, and reached a maximum on the third and fourth days; this was maintained until the seventh or eight day, after which the temperature gradually fell to normal. Relative bradycardia was present; tachycardia occurred only in the fatal cases. A second febrile attack was observed in some patients around the twelfth to the fourteenth days. Many patients suffered at onset from nausea and frequent, occasionally uncontrollable vomiting. Watery diarrhea was often observed, usually without admixtures of blood or mucous; in some cases extreme dehydration and kidney failure resulted.

All patients developed a characteristic, non-itching, maculopapulous rash on the fifth to eight day. It began in the face, and then progressed to the trunk and extremities. At first it consisted of tiny, sharply defined spots, often located around the hair follicles; then it developed into a rash consisting of middle-sized maculae, which merged to form a diffuse, dark-red erythema. Cutaneous petechiae were rare. The rash affected nearly the whole integument; it was especially marked on the scrotum and the greater labia. After its disappearance at about the end of the second week, a fine desquamation set in, which was especially conspicuous on the palms and soles.

At about the same stage, the majority of the patients developed an enanthema on the soft and hard palates; this consisted partly of tapioca-like blisters. About half of the patients had conjunctivitis and photophobia; no other changes in the eye were present.

Lymphadenitis was not infrequently observed in the nuchal, cervical, and axillary regions between the third and sixth days of illness. The lymph nodes were pea- to bean-sized, of soft consistency, and somewhat sensitive to pressure. In only one patient was the spleen palpable.

The central nervous system was affected in several patients. This was evident from their sullen, rebuffing, depressive behavior; they complained of par- and hyperaesthesia, myoclonism, and tremor. Some became confused, lapsed into unconsciousness, and died in cerebral coma, two of them with convulsions. One woman developed postinfectious myelitis with paralysis of both legs, and another a severe psychosis.

Around half of the patients exhibited marked hemorrhagic diathesis with spontaneous bleeding from the nose, gingiva, and gastrointestinal tract, as well as hematuria. All of the younger women showed genital bleeding independently of the menstrual cycle. Especially conspicuous were hematomas at sites of injection and heavy bleeding from the needle wounds. Prolonged thrombin and cephalin times were found in several patients, indicating a coagulopathy. EGBRING et al., 1971, have studied the bleeding mechanism in detail in guinea pigs (p. 132).

In nearly all patients the hemopoietic system was already disturbed in the first days of illness. A sudden, critical drop in the number of thrombocytes was observed, and marked leucopenia with an extreme shift to the left and release of immature cells. The red blood picture presented essentially no pathologic changes.

Most of the parenchymatous organs were affected. All patients had severe damage of the liver, evident from increased transaminase levels, which were extreme in some cases. It is interesting that neither jaundice nor hepatic coma developed. Electrocardiogram alterations were indicative of myocarditis; disturbances of rhythm and clinical signs of cardiac insufficiency were also present. The pancreas was affected in several patients, as was shown by the increased serum amylase values. Severely ill patients exhibited considerable kidney involvement with microhematuria, protein-, oligo-, and anuria, and retention of substances normally excreted in the urine. A brief episode of polyuria occurred in a few patients.

In differential diagnosis, rickettsioses and leptospiroses, typhoid and hemorrhagic fever were drawn into consideration, and particularly Russian spring-summer disease, Kyasanur Forest disease, Junin fever, Rift Valley fever, O'nynon-gnyong, Chikungunya (MARTINI et al., 1968 a), yellow fever and Oubangi hepatitis (STILLE et al., 1968). Although each of these diseases holds some features in common with the Marburg virus disease, important clinical differences are also present.

Among the laboratory findings, the hematologic changes were studied intensively (HAVEMANN and SCHMIDT, 1971). Leukopenia involving the neutrophils as well as the lymphocytes was most marked between the third and fifth days; in some cases their concentration dropped to less than $1000/mm^3$. The shift to the left consisted of up to 40 per cent stab cells, with a few promyelo-, metamyelo-, and myelocytes. By the second week the counts of neutrophils and lymphocytes had returned to normal, except for a few cases in which complications developed (bronchopneumonia, pleurisy) which involved excessive leukocytosis. In the third week monocytosis set in, followed in the fourth week by a lymphocytotic overshoot and moderate eosinophilia.

The shift to the left was accompanied by the frequent appearance of degenerative neutrophil cells in the peripheral blood; later, atypical lymphocytes, plasma cells, and immunoblasts were also found, but they never exceeded 15 per cent. This was the characteristic morphologic blood picture. Bone marrow punctures performed on three patients between the fifteenth and seventeenth days revealed corresponding changes in granulopoiesis, as well as an elevated number of immature megakaryocytes. The thrombocytes decreased continually from the first day of illness onward, reaching a minimum, in extreme cases below $10,000/mm^3$, between the sixth and twelfth days.

The characteristic liver enzymes (the transaminases SGOT and SGPT, glutamate dehydrase, sorbitol dehydrogenase, and glutamyl transpeptidase) were considerably increased in all cases, attaining a maximum at the start of the second week (MARTINI, 1969). In four of the five fatal cases studied the SGOT level exceeded 2500 U/l. The ratio of SGOT to SGPT reached a height of 7 : 1 in extreme cases. Bilirubin values were only slightly elevated, if at all. Serum alkaline phosphatase and creatinine phosphokinase remained normal. Creatine and urea increased only in case of anuria. Occasionally, enhanced amylase values were observed, as well as hypokalemia and lowering of the serum protein level to as little as 4.5 per cent.

The erythrocyte sedimentation rate seldom exceeded the upper normal range. Blood pressure showed a drop only ante exitum. At the height of the illness half of the patients exhibited ECG alterations (repolarization disturbances, dextrodelay, atrial fibrillation). A few lumbar punctures revealed a normal cell count with a normal to slightly elevated protein content.

Barring complications, the illness ran its course in fifteen to twenty days. Complications occurring at the peak included bronchopneumonia (five cases, one with pleurisy), pretibial edema (five cases), unilateral orchitis (three cases), postinfectious myelitis, and psychosis (one each).

Between the eighth and the sixteenth days after onset five men and two women died; they were between 19 and 64 years of age. This is a mortality rate of about 22 per cent. The immediate cause of death was cardiovascular failure, total anuria, or cerebral coma.

A total of five liver relapses with elevated transaminase values and slight fever were observed in the later stages of convalescence; one case was confirmed by demonstration of the pathogen in liver biopsy tissue. The convalescent period was very drawn out. Disturbances of the autonomic nervous system, such as an increased tendency to perspire and rapid fatigue were interpreted as late sequelae. Beyond this, the patients exhibited considerable loss of hair, and complained of stitches in the region of the liver and alcohol intolerance. Unilateral testicular atrophy occurred in five patients, accompanied in some by reduced libido and potency and oligospermia, but with normal ketosteroid levels.

The prognosis for recovery of the liver was good, as judged from the cases followed up with liver needle biopsies. Among twelve patients, only two showed somewhat elevated transaminases with slight liver cell reaction during the recovery period (4 to 31 days after becoming afebrile). All patients are under follow-up control, because of possible persistence of the infection.

Therapy was symptomatic. Antibiotics alone or in combination were without effect against viral manifestations; they are nevertheless to be recommended as prophylaxis against bacterial secondary infections. The most difficult problem was the treatment of the hemorrhagic diathesis. In order to bring the bleeding tendency under control, fresh blood, thrombocyte concentrates, fibrinogen, ε-aminocaproic acid, vitamin K, and the French preparation PPSB from the Centre National de Transfusion Sanguine were administered; the latter reduced the propensity to bleed for several hours at a time. In addition, supplementation of electrolytes, and in the presence of hypoproteinemia the administration of up to 30 g of human albumin daily, proved necessary. In spite of this, the plasma protein levels in some patients could be maintained at only 4 g per cent. In case of impairment of diuresis mannite (Osmofundin®) was infused; peritoneal dialysis was performed in anuria. Medication for the cardiovascular system was often required. Corticosteroids were ineffective in two patients in terminal stages. Antipyretics proved generally useful. The success of the use of convalescent sera in four cases in Frankfurt and Belgrade cannot be evaluated, because a few less severe courses were observed even where no serum was injected.

B. Pathology

The pathologic anatomy of the Marburg virus disease was studied intensively on five patients, including one woman, who had died between the eighth and the sixteenth day after onset (GEDIGK et al., 1968; 1971; BECHTELSHEIMER, 1968; KORB et al., 1968). The different durations of the illness prior to death made it possible to make inferences concerning the chronology of the morphologic changes during the course of the disease.

The macroscopic findings were notably similar in all cases, but they did not bring much information. All patients had edematous swelling of the brain with hyperemia of the leptomeninges, such as occurs in cases of central nervous death. In addition, considerable hemorrhaging was occasionally apparent in the skin, mucous membranes, and parenchymatous organs. In most of the fatal cases the stomach and parts of the intestine were filled with blood. Petechiae could be seen in the mucosa of the stomach and the small intestine. In no case was the liver smaller than normal; instead of the normal lobular markings, a fine, partly yellowish-grayish-reddish, partly brown-reddish mottling was apparent. The gall bladders were dilated and engorged. No jaundice and no indication of disturbed bilirubin excretion were present. The spleen was enlarged in only two patients; swollen lymph nodes, in contrast, were generally observed, particularly in the abdomen and the lung hili. The kidneys exhibited cloudy swelling. A livid-bluish discoloration of the scrotum or labia was noticed. Two patients had broncho-pneumonia. Cardiac dilatation was evident in all cases. These macroscopic findings are not sufficiently characteristic to permit diagnosis of any definite disease.

Histologically, signs of hemorrhagic diathesis were conspicuous; this must be considered in connection with the thrombocytopenia which had been observed clinically. In addition, most organs, except for the lungs, brain, bones, and skeletal muscle, exhibited focal necroses without substantial inflammatory reaction. The necrobiotic processes corresponded in their staining reactions to coagulation necroses, and were located for the most part in the parenchyma of the liver, spleen, lymph nodes, testes, ovaries, and pancreas. Kidneys, adenohypophysis, thyroid gland, suprarenals, and skin were affected to a considerably lesser extent.

The greatly elevated serum transaminase values indicated severe damage of the liver, corresponding to hepatitis, the nature and course of which stimulated special interest (KORB et al., 1969; BECHTELSHEIMER et al., 1970; 1971). The earliest changes could not be studied in man, because the victims died only at the peak of the illness or as remission was beginning. The initial stages in the development were studied in experiments on guinea pigs (p. 114). Later changes were studied in liver biopsies from fifteen patients, taken between the 13th and the 39th days after onset; these findings were compared with those on infected guinea pigs.

Necroses of single liver cells, as well as of groups of cells, occurred irregularly scattered throughout all lobular zones, along with necroses of individual Kupffer cells. The reticular fibers remained intact. A peak was reached in the second week, after which rapid disintegration and resorption took place. The necroses were characterized by partly homogeneous, partly plaque-like transformation of the cytoplasm, as well as by a positive PAS reaction and an enhanced affinity for eosin. In the vicinity of these changes numerous mitotic hepatocytes and occasional infiltration of lymphoidocytes were observed. In all fatal cases there was a diffuse fatty degeneration with fine to middle-sized droplets. In the vicinity of large necroses considerable proliferation of the Kupffer cells was found. The defects were replaced by regenerated liver cells. At no point was there significant cholestasia or siderosis.

Subsequent changes were found to depend upon the degree of damage to the liver tissue. In cases in which the transaminase values remained below 500 mU/ml, only noncharacteristic alterations were observed later; in those having higher enzyme levels, single cell necroses, diffuse fatty degeneration of the liver, and occasional intralobular fibrotic zones could be demonstrated. Transformative processes, i. e., postnecrotic cirrhosis, were not found. In spite of extensive necrosis, restitution of the structure of the liver is considered likely. The hepatitis caused by the Marburg virus showed combinations and effects which differ distinctly from those of the classical hepatitis forms, yellow fever, or other hemorrhagic fevers (BECHTELSHEIMER et al., 1970; 1971).

Likewise characteristic of the Marburg virus disease is the plasma-cellular, monocytoidal transformation of the lymphatic tissue. Besides total or partial follicular necroses and perifollicular hemorrhages, the red pulp of the spleen and the medulla of the lymph nodes contained conspicuously few cells and dense deposits of granulated, eosinophilic, PAS-positive material, possibly thrombocyte aggregations. Small nodules consisting of reticular cells developed instead of follicular necroses. In later stages, almost cell-free, hyalinized regions were found to remain. Even later, increasingly plasma-cellular, monocytoid infiltration occurred in the mucous membranes of the stomach and intestines; these might possibly have been evidence of an immunologic process.

Aside from interstitial edema and hemorrhaging, the testes exhibited extensive necrosis with destruction of the seminiferous tubules. Concentric necroses were also observed in the ovaries, especially in the granulosa layer of the secondary follicles. Necroses in the pancreas affected the islets of Langerhans more than the excretory portions. Without exception the kidneys showed signs of severe tubular insufficiency. The minor or entirely inapparent heart muscle damage in spite of the presence of interstitial edema was surprising; the latter was therefore interpreted less as a result of myocarditis than as a consequence of increased permeability of the capillary walls.

Many patients suffered from clouding of consciousness, either temporarily or as a transition to coma, indicating involvement of the central nervous system. This clinical impression was confirmed in detailed neuropathologic studies (BECHTELSHEIMER et al., 1968; JACOB and SOLCHER, 1968; JACOB, 1971). The latter were based in three of the five fatal cases in Marburg on whole-brain sections including the cerebral and cerebellar hemispheres, the basal ganglia, and the brain stem down to the medulla oblongata. From the other two patients only selected parts of the brain were available.

Common to all cases was congestion of the cerebral and meningeal vessels, accompanied by perivascular bleeding, which was of minor extent in some cases. In three patients glial nodule encephalitis developed in the gray and the white matter of all portions of the brain down to the medulla oblongata, affecting some of the roots of the spinal nerves as well. Besides this, occasional lymphocytic-perivascular foci of inflammation were described. The glial nodules consisted predominantly of glious cells, but also contained a few histiocytic-epithelioid elements. They varied in size from a few cells to larger cell aggregations having a diameter of 300 mμ. According to their cellular composition, density, structure, and arrangement they were divided into three types. Necrotic changes were absent. Noteworthy were localized aggregations of nodules in the cerebellar cortex, as well as in the cerebral cortex and the white matter; their extent depended upon the duration of the illness.

No glial nodules were found in the patients who died after a single day of unconsciousness; however, considerable vascular congestion with seroerythrocytic diapedesis was evident. In one case massive bleeding had taken place in the corpus callosum. The generalized hemorrhagic diathesis was probably responsible for the bleeding in the central nervous system.

The neuropathologic events were similar to those in numerous other encephalitides, especially in typhus and arbovirus infections. Beside the large number of common features, however, clear differences exist. The encephalitides in the diseases mentioned exhibit a greater complexity; in contrast to the "pure" glial nodule encephalitis of the Marburg virus disease, they are characterized by intensive signs of inflammation in the mesenchymal tissue, destruction of neurons by neurophagia, focal necroses, and spongy degeneration.

A regular finding consisted of round, basophilic cytoplasmic bodies with a diameter of 1–4 μ. They were especially numerous within or in the vicinity of necroses, in cell remains, and in phagocytes, but were also evident in intact liver and kidney cells. Eosinophilic inclusions, surrounded by a narrow cytoplasmic halo, were also observed occasionally; their nature is not yet understood. Nevertheless, their high DNA content suggests that they are nuclear fragments. Exact fluorescence-serologic and electron microscopic studies are still lacking.

Among the causes of death the damage to the central nervous system certainly was an important factor. In addition, toxemia due to liver damage and tubular insufficiency of the kidneys was also present. Failure of the cardiovascular system was also involved. The role of the hemorrhagic diathesis and the diarrhea cannot be evaluated on the basis of the anatomic findings. Suppurative hemorrhagic bronchopneumonia was the cause of death in one case. Although the Marburg virus disease is not characterized by any specific pathologic-anatomic alterations, the extent, combination, and pattern of distribution of these changes in the various organs justify classifying it as a disease which was previously unknown.

C. Diagnosis

1. Isolation of the Virus

During the febrile phase the Marburg virus was found in blood, serum, and organ tissues (liver, spleen, kidney, lung, brain) of all patients (SIEGERT et al., 1967 a, b; 1968 a, b, c; SMITH et al., 1967; KUNZ et al., 1968 a; MAY and KNOTHE, 1968; KISSLING et al., 1968; SIMPSON et al., 1968 a, b; MALHERBE and STRICKLAND-CHOLMLEY, 1968; STOJKOVIĆ et al., 1968; 1971). Besides guinea pigs, primary simian cell cultures and BHK-21 cells also proved suitable for the cultivation of the Marburg virus.

In addition, the agent could be demonstrated during the acute phase in two of six throat washings and in one of four urine samples, but not in five stool samples. The virus was clearly less concentrated than in blood; it was, in fact, barely discernable. Outside of the febrile stage no viremia could be detected, but virus was still isolated from a liver needle biopsy cylinder during a liver relapse, and in the semen of a long-term excretor (SIEGERT et al., 1968 b, c).

No diagnostic experience with monkeys which have acquired the disease under natural conditions has yet been made. In experimentally infected animals, as in man, the agent was found during the acute stage in blood, organ material, saliva, and urine (SIMPSON et al., 1968 a; HAAS et al., 1968 b). Its detection in a rectal swabbing was most likely due to contamination with blood.

Rapid clarification of the etiology is of prime importance in a disease so dangerous to man and monkeys alike. The high concentration of virus in blood and liver during the febrile stage permits quick diagnosis by direct demonstration of the antigen and the virus (SIEGERT, 1969; SIEGERT and SLENCZKA, 1971).

Virus antigen in blood from patients was made visible by means of immunofluorescence, where it appeared in thick drops as extracellular aggregations with
a diameter of 1–10 μ, as well as in smears of liver biopsy material and of semen.
The impression gained was that of extruded inclusions. All findings were corroborated in experiments on guinea pigs (SIEGERT et al., 1968 b, c). In monkeys
the infection could be detected histologically as early as the fourth day after
infection, even before development of symptoms (OEHLERT, 1971). As in other
subjects, predominantly intracytoplasmic inclusions of antigen were found in
liver, spleen, and lymph nodes (HAAS et al., 1968 b).

Direct electron microscopic demonstration of the virus was possible after
centrifugation (40,000 × g) of serum or plasma onto carrier films, using the method
of MÜLLER (1969), and in thin sections of liver. The unusual size, the pleomorphism,
and the structure of the viria are so characteristic that no doubt occurred as to the
identity of the pathogen (SIEGERT et al., 1967 b; PETERS and MÜLLER, 1968).

Ambiguous or negative findings in rapid diagnosis must be followed up by
isolation experiments using guinea pigs and cell culture systems. If the animals
develop a fever within ten days after intraperitoneal administration of the
material under study, the specifity of the illness must be examined. This can be
done by reinfection or by demonstration of antibodies in convalescent guinea pigs.
An additional possibility is the demonstration of specific inclusion bodies in liver
tissue smears from passage animals using immunofluorescence (SIEGERT et al.,
1967 b; 1968).

No cytopathic effect was observed in cell cultures (p. 126), especially in the
first passage. In primary simian kidney or Vero cell cultures, however, antigen
inclusions were apparent as early as the third day; they increase considerably in
size and number until the seventh day (SLENCZKA et al., 1968; MALHERBE and
STRICKLAND-CHOLMLEY, 1968).

2. Serodiagnosis

Antibody was likewise shown to be present in all patients. The neutralization
test using guinea pigs and cell cultures is not suitable for routine diagnosis (p. 107),
although proof of increasing titers was obtained in some individual cases (SIEGERT
et al., 1968 a; SLENCZKA, 1969 a).

The complement fixation test, in contrast, has proved valuable. SMITH et al.
(1967) were the first to observe increasing titers of complement-fixing antibodies
specific for antigen from infected guinea pig organs in several patients. Because
of slight cross reactions between normal guinea pig control antigen and normal
human sera, HOFMANN and KUNZ (1969 a) regarded only titers exceeding 1 : 8 as
positive. The highest titers reported by STOJKOVIĆ et al. (1971) were 1 : 32 to
1 : 64, and were reached during the third week, at the latest in the fourth.

It must be taken into consideration that virus antigen derived from organs of
infected animals contains more or less large amounts of nonspecific antigenic
material (p. 108). Thus, like control antigen from normal guinea pig liver, it frequently reacts with normal sera. Human immune sera also often show nonspecific
reactions with normal antigen which are just as strong as those with virus antigen.
Considerable variations were found in the titers in different samples from the same
healthy person, simulating "titer jumps" between two serum samples. For this

reason use of viral antigen derived from animal tissues presents problems in the evaluation of "positive" results (SLENCZKA et al., 1970; SLENCZKA and WOLFF, 1971).

Because of its greater specificity, SLENCZKA et al. (1970, 1971) recommend complement-fixing antigen from "chronically" infected Vero carrier cells. They used such antigen to study the behavior of the antibody titers in 22 patients. The increase occurred within the first three weeks after onset. Between the fourth and eighth weeks the highest levels were attained; these still persisted six months later. Considerable individual variations in titer during the course of the disease were observed in three patients. With a single exception the complement-fixing antibodies were still clearly demonstrable after about two years. Serodiagnosis proved to be just as reliable as demonstrations of virus.

V. Epidemiology and Epizootiology

The nature and distribution of the disease were not immediately recognized for various reasons. Only after they had been ill for several days did the patients seek the advice of their family physicians, most of whom initially suspected only common infectious illnesses (e. g., gastroenteritis or angina). Delays in the mail, vacations, and the five-day work week contributed an additional two to six days to the delay (HENNESSEN et al., 1968; NITTNER, 1971). The clinical peculiarities and the common source of infection first became apparent when several severely ill monkey caretakers were brought to the university hospitals in Marburg/Lahn and Frankfurt/Main (MARTINI et al., 1968 a; STILLE et al., 1968). Onset of the disease in each of the 31 patients is tabulated in Fig. 20. According to the mode of exposure, three groups can be distinguished, for which the mean incubation periods differ by one and two weeks, respectively (HENNESSEN et al., 1968; HENNESSEN, 1969; 1971).

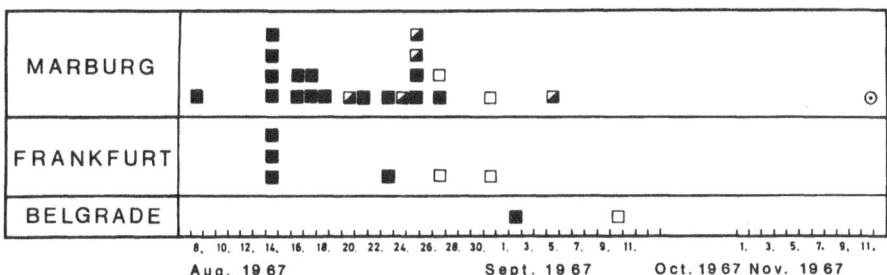

Fig. 20. Onset of Marburg virus disease in 31 cases. [Taken from HENNESSEN et al., MARTINI et al., STILLE et al., Dtsch. med. Wschr. 93, Nr. 12 a (1968).]

The first group of patients to fall ill was also the largest. It consisted of persons who had had direct contact with blood and organs of monkeys, and comprised two veterinarians, who had performed post mortem dissections of the monkeys, and 18 monkey caretakers, whose duties included feeding and catching the animals, plus giving electric shocks, performing injection anaesthesia, phlebotomies, ventral nephrectomies, skull trepanations, post mortems, disposing of the cadavers, cleaning the animal quarters and equipment, and carrying out disinfection and sterilization procedures (HENNESSEN et al., 1968).

When performing aseptic phlebotomies or removing organs from the monkeys the personnel wore the usual protective clothing, with gloves and face masks. In the other duties the personal protection measures remained more or less incomplete. During cleaning no masks or gloves were worn, and the forearms were likewise unprotected. Thus the possibility of contact with monkey blood was given in every primary case of the illness. Twenty of the 29 persons exposed in this manner fell ill. The great risk of infection is not surprising in view of the unusually high concentrations of Marburg virus in blood and organs of infected monkeys (HAAS et al., 1968 b; PETERS and MÜLLER, 1968; SIMPSON et al., 1968 a; SIMPSON, 1969 d). The extent to which infectious products of excretion of the animals were involved is not known. The significance of direct contact with the animals was emphasized by the fact that four caretakers who were responsible for the animals only on weekends, when no bleeding or removal of organs were performed, remained unaffected.

The second group consisted of five laboratory workers who had more or less close contact with simian organs or cell culture material (HENNESSEN et al., 1968; HENNESSEN, 1969; 1971). Ten of their colleagues remained healthy despite similar exposure. The duties of the laboratory personnel included fetching the kidneys from the animal operating room, preparing tissue cultures from them, and washing the glassware and instruments, whereby in one case injury was caused by broken glass. Only the setting up of cell cultures was performed under sterile conditions with face masks and gloves; personal protection measures were neglected when cleaning. Therefore this group, too, had ample possibility of contact with blood and cell material from monkeys. In contrast, no illnesses occurred in three institutions which received monkey kidneys during this period from one of the affected vaccine producers; nor have any cases appeared in any of the twelve institutes in which subsequent experiments with the Marburg virus were carried out.

As has been described elsewhere (p. 130), several laboratory technicians contracted infections by contact with cell cultures derived from monkey kidney tissue. For this reason MAASS et al. (1969) pursued the epidemiologically important question of whether the Marburg virus can be demonstrated in cell cultures from experimentally infected cercopithecans, and whether its presence has an effect on the growth of the culture cells in vitro. The development of the cell monolayer was not different from that of noninfected control cultures. It was possible to establish subcultures in which the Marburg virus was likewise present. Treatment with trypsin had no effect on the infection. Cellular infection induced an incomplete CPE and could be recognized on the basis of eosinophilic inclusions, which varied considerably in number according to the animal donor. The antigen could be visualized by immunofluorescence and the virus itself by electron microscopy. The cell culture supernatant was found to contain virus titers of between 10^{-2} and $10^{-4.7}$/ml.

The third category comprised the largest group of exposed persons, but their exact number is unknown. Six of them contracted the disease, all from patients (MARTINI et al., 1968 a; STILLE et al., 1968; TODOROVITCH et al., 1971). The mode and the time of infection in the cases of two attending physicians is known exactly, for they unfortunately suffered scratches from injection needles through their rubber gloves after having taken blood samples. One injury showed an inflammatory reaction. A laboratory technician and a post-mortem technician likewise came into direct contact with patients' blood. In the case of a nurse it seems likely that she acquired the infection by way of contaminated air or contact with excreta, for as far as is known she had had no contact with blood.

Exposure in the household and family milieu remained without consequences, with a single exception; this involved the wife of a patient who had recovered seven weeks earlier. It was then discovered that her husband had continued to excrete the Marburg virus, and had infected his wife via his semen. The vaginal infection was presumably facilitated by mucosal erosion following total hysterectomy for carcinoma of the uterus and irradiation (MARTINI and SCHMIDT, 1968; SIEGERT et al., 1968 c). The existence of latent infections among the exposed persons could be excluded by serologic studies (SLENCZKA et al., 1970).

The human contact infections entered through lesions of the skin and mucous membranes. According to laboratory experience, the intact skin seems to provide an effective barrier (SHU et al., 1968). The infectious materials involved were blood from the febrile phase and semen; throat secretions and urine, in contrast, probably played only a relatively minor role because of their low concentrations of virus (SIEGERT et al., 1968 c). The chain of infection terminated at the latest after two human passages. All infections resulted in clinical manifestation.

The simultaneous outbreak of the disease in Frankfurt and in Marburg was traced to common imported stocks of monkeys of the species Cercopithecus aethiops from Uganda. Nevertheless, this is supported only by indirect evidence based on the exposure and incubation periods of the patients. Animals of the implicated shipments were no longer available for diagnosis of the pathogen. Agents which proved pathogenic for guinea pigs, however, were discovered in Frankfurt in a cell culture frozen at this time, and in tissues derived from cercopithecans which had arrived later in Marburg (HENNESSEN et al., 1968; ROBIN et al., 1971); they induced a febrile reaction in guinea pigs and could be propagated in passages. Unfortunately, they were never identified serologically or in electron microscopy. The two cases of the disease in Belgrade were likewise traced to shipments from the same animal catching station in Uganda. Antibody was found three months later in 36 of 41 cercopithecans, but its specificity is subject to question (STOJKOVIĆ et al., 1971) (p. 108). HENNESSEN (1969, 1971) found it necessary to assume at least five different sources of infection involving a minimum of ten infected monkeys in order to explain the twenty cases affecting the veterinarians and animal caretakers in Marburg. The cases in Frankfurt must have involved at least another two infectious animals, and those in Belgrade one affected monkey. Four shipments were determined as possible sources; they had arrived in Europe between July

20th and August 10th, 1967, and comprised a total of 500—600 animals. Their distribution to the affected institutions was quite various. Frankfurt received only 10 per cent, and this small number in two batches. It is hardly likely that all the monkeys were infectious from the start; in that case an increased mortality would be expected, which was reported only from Belgrade (STOJKOVIĆ *et al.*, 1971). Presumably the infection spread during the course of three weeks in the groups of monkeys kept in quarantine for 25 days in Belgrade and in Marburg for up to 29 days (HENNESSEN *et al.*, 1968). The animals probably became contagious five to eight days after exposure. Even if we assume this minimal time, the first monkeys must have acquired the infection before their arrival. Prompt recognition is difficult; experiments have shown that the symptoms, which are nonspecific in nature, develop only shortly preceding death (p. 111). Even highly infectious monkeys with large amounts of virus in blood, urine, and saliva can appear healthy; infectivity can even precede the febrile stage. It is unknown whether protracted excretion occurs in monkeys.

Our knowledge of the propagation of the Marburg virus among monkeys is based solely on experimental data on *Cercopithecus*, *Macaca mulatta*, and *Saimiri sciureus* (SIMPSON *et al.*, 1968 a, b; SIMPSON, 1969 d; HAAS *et al.*, 1968 a, b, c; HAAS and MAASS, 1971). In captivity transmission probably occurred by means of smear infections of animals occupying the same cages. This is not surprising, as during the febrile phase not only blood and saliva, but also urine and bloody stools are highly infectious. In cases involving several monkeys in separate cages in the same room, aerogenic transmission is suspected. Arthropods were hardly a likely factor in spreading the disease within the animal quarters. It is nevertheless conceivable that they are involved in transmission under natural conditions, for multiplication of the agent has been observed to occur in *Aedes aegypti* (KUNZ *et al.*, 1968 b; HOFMANN and KUNZ, 1968; HOFMANN *et al.*, 1969).

Human cases have been reported only in the Federal Republic of Germany and in Yugoslavia, although numerous shipments of monkeys from the same dealer were sent simultaneously from Uganda to the USA, Italy, Japan, Sweden, and Switzerland (WILLIAMS *et al.*, 1968). This prompted a search for peculiar epidemiologic circumstances. No pertinent evidence was found among diseases occurring in Central Africa (KAPLAN, 1969; WILLIAMS *et al.*, 1968). It was found, however, that in view of a considerable increase in demand the time elapsed between capture, shipment, and use of the monkeys in experiments had shortened considerably since 1967 (HENDERSON *et al.*, 1971). In addition, because of the Near East crisis, the animals were flown to Germany and Yugoslavia via London instead of directly as before. There, during layovers of from 9 to 36 hours, the monkeys were kept in quarters where they had the possibility of contact with 48 species of animals from all over the world (HENNESSEN *et al.*, 1968; WILLIAMS *et al.*, 1968). The otherwise usual isolation of the monkeys from the other animals could not be enforced because of overfilling of the facilities. In particular, the contact with non-european finches and two langurs *(Presbytis)* from Ceylon have been mentioned, one of which died (HENNESSEN *et al.*, 1968). No antibody was found in the surviving langur (SIMPSON *et al.*, 1968 a). Nevertheless it seems more likely that the reservoir of the Marburg virus is in the native habitat of the monkeys in Africa. Monkeys themselves did not seem to be the probable natural reservoir of the virus, since in spite of their widespread use in experiments transmission of this hemorrhagic fever in laboratories has not been otherwise observed. The fact that all infections of monkeys proved lethal under experimental conditions, even after minimal dosages, also supports this contention. For this reason it came as a great surprise when seroepidemiologic studies indicated a wide distribution of the Marburg virus, not only among monkeys from Central Africa, but also among those from Asia and America.

Seroepidemiologic investigations were based almost exclusively on the detection of complement-fixing antibody in the most various species of monkeys from three continents. Other species and humans coming into contact with monkeys were studied only occasionally. In most cases the antigens used were derived from infected guinea pig organs (p. 108). The findings are inconsistent.

Whereas SIMPSON et al. (1968 a) found no complement-fixing antibody in 201 blood samples from vervet monkeys from Uganda, reports coming from the Special Studies Laboratory, NCDC (1968) indicated that of 129 African green monkeys from Ethiopia, Kenya, and Uganda, 50 per cent reacted positively. No differences were found between animals imported into the USA and those studied immediately following capture. The same percentage of antibody carriers was also determined in a limited number of chimpanzees, gorillas, and orangutans. STOJ-KOVIĆ et al. (1968, 1971) found positive reactions among most of 41 cercopithecans three months after their arrival in Belgrade, but in only two out of 49 cercopithecans from Kenya. Using KISSLING's antigen, KALTER et al. (1969) was unable to detect antibody in Africans, laboratory personnel, gorillas, orangutans, gibbons, or marmosets. In contrast, some cynomolgus and rhesus monkey sera, and all sera from chimpanzees, baboons, African green monkeys, patas, and talapoins exhibited varying titers of complement-fixing antibody. It was especially emphasized that under similar experimental conditions baboons and chimpanzees which had been born in captivity were free of antibody.

Since this hemorrhagic fever had never been observed before, either in humans or in animals, WILLIAMS et al. (1968) and HENDERSON et al. (1971) undertook field studies in the areas where the monkeys exported to Europe had been captured. They performed isolation tests and serologic studies involving monkey trappers and traders, monkeys, and rodents. The pathogen could not be demonstrated in any organ or serum samples from the animals. Of 207 monkey sera obtained mostly from Cercopithecus aethiops between August and October 1967, 36 per cent reacted "positively" with viral antigen derived from guinea pig liver which had been absorbed with hamster liver powder. Only those titers were considered positive which were at least four times as high as those with normal control antigen. Increases in titer were observed in nine cercopithecans. It was concluded from the increasing percentage of animals showing complement-fixing antibody that the Marburg virus or an agent related to it circulated during these months in the regions of Lake Kyoga and Entebbe. Of 79 monkey trappers, none of whom reported having had any unusual illness, three had complement-fixing antibody titers of 1 : 8; two of these also reacted positively in neutralization tests. This was interpreted as proof of the occurrence of the infection among humans in Uganda. Out of 80 rats one positive sample was found; thus rodents might also be worthy of suspicion as virus reservoirs.

In order to determine whether an association exists between the pathogen and African monkeys, KALTER (1971) extended his serologic studies to include, in particular, monkeys from Asia and from America. Its occurrence in Africa was suggested principally by the high percentage of positive reactions among baboons (blood samples taken immediately upon capture), and by the fact that positive titers had been found less frequently in monkeys from Asia and the New World. Thus, the conspicuously high percentage of positive findings among Japanese macaques was all the more surprising. Contact with African monkeys is cited as being responsible for this, since sero-conversions have been observed in captivity and in SFRE animals. It does not seem consistent with the frequent findings of antibody in monkeys, however, that neither illness nor excessive mortality was observed, as would have been expected on the basis of experimental experience. With such widespread contamination it is also difficult to imagine why no cases have occurred until now involving humans having close contact with monkeys.

For this reason scepticism was expressed regarding the specificity of the antigen used in the complement fixation tests, and the interpretation of the findings. To be sure, STRICKLAND-CHOLMLEY and MALHERBE (1970, 1971) agreed with KALTER et al. (1969) that a high percentage of monkey sera (61 per cent) reacted with antigen from infectious guinea pig organs; but in comparative studies using antigen from infectious monkey liver only 7 of 292 baboons (Papio ursinus) and vervet monkeys (Cercopithecus aethiops pygerythrus) which had reacted with KISSLING's antigen were found to be positive. They questioned the specificity of the findings obtained with this antigen because of the occurrence of cross reactions with liver antigen. They concluded, that the "United States antigen" probably contained a second component not specific for Marburg virus, which fixed complement in tests on simian sera. The authors are convinced that the Marburg virus is absent among the two species studied in South Africa, or occurs at most only to a limited extent. HENDERSON et al. (1971) point out the possibility that the antibodies might not only have been directed against the Marburg virus but simultaneously against a less pathogenic related virus which circulated in Uganda at the same time.

On the basis of detailed comparisons of specificity of various antigens used in complement fixation tests, SLENCZKA et al. (1970, 1971) have developed a cell culture antigen from infected Vero carrier cells which fulfills all requirements of specificity and effectiveness (p. 108). With these preparations no complement-fixing antibody could be demonstrated in any of the 136 monkeys from Uganda and South Africa, or in 25 serum samples which had been found positive by other teams in preliminary tests. Likewise negative was the detection of antibody by means of indirect immunofluorescence. Thus, as has been indicated, it seems probable that the supposed discovery of antibody was based on nonspecific reactions. For this reason it seems inappropriate to refer to the Marburg virus as a simian virus so long as its origin remains unclear. Determination of the virus reservoir is one of the most important tasks yet to be accomplished. It is not impossible that a unique chance event is involved; this is suggested by the morphologic similarity of the Marburg virus to a whole roster of plant viruses.

VI. Control and Prevention

The sudden and surprising outbreak of the disease confronted the institutions and health authorities affected with demanding responsibilities. Measures had to be introduced to control a still unidentified pathogen, the origin and transmission of which were not known. Wearing of protective clothing with gloves was immediately ordered, not only for work with the monkeys, but also during all preparation and cleaning. After the suspicion had become stronger that the source of infection lay in several particular shipments of monkeys (Cercopithecus aethiops), all stocks of monkeys were gassed to death, all cell cultures derived from monkey tissues destroyed, and the animal quarters and laboratories disinfected. Thereafter no new cases of the illness occurred among the animal caretakers or laboratory personnel (HENNESSEN et al., 1968; HENNESSEN 1969; 1971).

The patients were placed in quarantine stations and cared for by volunteers. In spite of precautionary measures, contact infections appeared, due to unfortunate circumstances (MARTINI et al., 1968; STILLE et al., 1968). Most of the patients were released from quarantine ten to fourteen days after complete recovery. Because of the frequency of orchitis, the men were advised to exercise sexual restraint (MARTINI and SCHMIDT, 1968). Laboratory personnel in the clinics and in the microbiology and pathology institutes worked under the usual conditions of personal protection, which proved to be adequate.

The possibility of spreading of the disease to the general population was met with comprehensive antiepidemic measures (NITTNER, 1971). All persons who had had contact with monkey material or with the patients (over 100 persons) were examined daily at their homes by public health physicians. This made it possible to spot all subsequent cases immediately. Exposed persons were temporarily forbidden to work in food stores or restaurants, go to school, or donate blood. General practitioners were informed via circulars of the clinical picture and the particular problems involved. Frequent press conferences proved especially valuable in preventing panic among the public.

The events in Marburg, Frankfurt, and Belgrade resulted in a total ban on importation and shipment of monkeys (Simiae) and lemurs (Prosimiae) in the Federal Republic of Germany and in Yugoslavia, so that no experiments with monkeys were possible, and no simian kidney cells were available for the production of vaccines or for virus diagnostics. Legal provisions concerning importation and handling of monkeys were considerably expanded and made more stringent, in order to prevent the recurrence of a similar outbreak (ANDERS, 1971; SCHUMACHER, 1971). Similarly, the WHO has proposed recommendations for the capture, transport, ex- and importation, quarantine, veterinary inspection, and trade of monkeys, for the purpose of improving the health of laboratory primates in the future (BEVERIDGE, 1971).

Reservoir and distribution of the Marburg virus are still unknown. For this reason the risk of future outbreaks cannot yet be determined. Even though the experience gained so far would make the risk seem to be small, all imported monkeys should nevertheless be regarded as potential sources of infection for man, regardless of whether species from Africa or other continents are involved. All

10b

monkey species examined to date have proved to be highly susceptible, so that they may be considered theoretically as possible carriers.

The six-week quarantine period now required should reduce the risk, for the infection can be counted on to manifest its presence by way of increased mortality rates. The etiology can then be cleared up on the basis of the characteristic histopathologic changes in the organs and by means of virologic studies.

Precautionary measures are necessary wherever monkeys are kept; in all sorts of experiments involving monkeys; in use of organ material in cell cultures, for transplantation, and for production of vaccines; and in caring for patients with the Marburg monkey disease.

In order to preclude direct contact, protective clothing with rubber gloves and a face mask must be worn. In addition, strict measures for the disinfection of excreta and of the air (UV lamp, disinfectant sprays) are necessary. Combatting insects and vermin would also seem advisable, although it is not yet known whether arthropods can serve as vectors.

Several precautionary measures have been introduced into the process of vaccine production in order to prevent contamination with the Marburg virus (BONIN, 1971). Because of its size, the pathogen can be eliminated from vaccines or cultural media by filtration. A guinea pig test was already in use for demonstration of tubercle bacilli; the fever measurements had only to be extended to cover the first four weeks. For detection of the virus, an additional test has been introduced in Germany, in which the body temperatures of five guinea pigs are measured over a period of two to three weeks. Blind transfers of blood, liver, or spleen tissue to five additional animals are then made, which in case of febrile reaction must be followed by histopathologic and virologic examination. In cell cultures which show no cytopathic effect the infection can be recognized by the presence of cytoplasmic inclusions.

References

ALMEIDA, J. D., A. P. WATERSON, D. M. BERRY, and L. H. TURNER: Structures associated with leptospires possibly relevant to the Marburg agent. Lancet i, 235—237 (1969).

ALMEIDA, J. D., A. P. WATERSON, and D. I. H. SIMPSON: Morphology and morphogenesis of the Marburg agent. In: Marburg Virus Disease, pp. 84—97. Springer-Verlag, Berlin-Heidelberg-New York, 1971.

ANDERS, W.: The vervet monkey disease, protection against occupational hazards. In: Marburg Virus Disease, pp. 220—222. Springer-Verlag, Berlin-Heidelberg-New York, 1971.

BECHTELSHEIMER, H.: Die pathologische Anatomie der ,,Marburg-Virus"-Krankheit. Habilitationsschrift Marburg/Lahn (1968).

BECHTELSHEIMER, H., H. JACOB und H. SOLCHER: Zur Neuropathologie der durch grüne Meerkatzen (Cercopithecus aethiops) übertragenen Infektionskrankheiten in Marburg. Dtsch. med. Wschr. **93**, 602—604 (1968), German Med. Monthly **XIV**, 10—12 (1969).

BECHTELSHEIMER, H., G. KORB und P. GEDIGK: Die ,,Marburg-Virus"-Hepatitis. Virchows Arch. path. Anat. **351**, 273—290 (1970).

BECHTELSHEIMER, H., G. KORB, and P. GEDIGK: Marburg virus hepatitis. In: Marburg Virus Disease, pp. 62—67. Springer-Verlag, Berlin-Heidelberg-New York, 1971.

BEVERIDGE, W. I. B.: W.H.O. draft recommendations for the supply, safe-handling, and use of non-human primates for biomedical purposes. In: Marburg Virus Disease, p. 226. Springer-Verlag, Berlin-Heidelberg-New York, 1971.

BONIN, O: Marburg virus: consequences for the manufacture and control of virus vaccines. In: Marburg Virus Disease, pp. 227—230. Springer-Verlag, Berlin-Heidelberg-New York, 1971.

BOWEN, E. T. W., D. I. H. SIMPSON, W. F. BRIGHT, I. ZLOTNIK, and D. M. R. HOWARD: Vervet monkey disease: studies on some physical and chemical properties of the causative agent. Brit. J. exp. Path. 50, 400—407 (1969).

CARTER, G. B., and W. F. BRIGHT: Immunfluorescent study of the vervet-monkey-disease agent. Lancet ii, 913—914 (1968).

CASALS, J.: see SIEGERT et al. (1968 b).

CASALS, J.: Absence of serological relationship between the Marburg virus and some arboviruses. In: Marburg Virus Disease, pp. 98—104. Springer-Verlag, Berlin-Heidelberg-New York, 1971.

CHUMAKOV, M. P.: personal communication (1968).

DAVID-WEST, T. S., and N. A. LABZOFFSKY: Studies on the site of replication of vesicular stomatitis virus. Arch. ges. Virusforsch. 24, 30—47 (1968).

EGBRING, R., W. SLENCZKA, and G. BALTZER: Clinical manifestations and mechanism of the haemorrhagic diathesis in Marburg virus disease. In: Marburg Virus Disease, pp. 41—49. Springer-Verlag, Berlin-Heidelberg-New York, 1971.

GEDIGK, P., H. BECHTELSHEIMER und G. KORB: Die pathologische Anatomie der „Marburg-Virus"-Krankheit (sog. „Marburger Affenkrankheit"). Dtsch. med. Wschr. 93, 590—601 (1968), German Med. Monthly XIV, 58—67 (1969).

GEDIGK, P., H. BECHTELSHEIMER, and G. KORB: Pathologic anatomy of the Marburg virus disease. In: Marburg Virus Disease, pp. 50—53. Springer-Verlag, Berlin-Heidelberg-New York, 1971.

HAAS, R., and G. MAASS: Experimental infection of monkeys with the Marburg virus. In: Marburg Virus Disease, pp. 136—143. Springer-Verlag, Berlin-Heidelberg-New York, 1971.

HAAS, R., G. MAASS und W. OEHLERT: Untersuchungen zur Tierpathogenität eines von Cercopithecus aethiops übertragenen menschenpathogenen Erregers. Med. Klinik 63, 1359—1363 (1968 a).

HAAS, R., G. MAASS, J. MÜLLER und W. OEHLERT: Experimentelle Infektionen von Cercopithecus aethiops mit dem Erreger des Frankfurt-Marburg-Syndroms (FMS). Z. med. Mikrobiol. Immunol. 154, 210—220 (1968 b).

HAAS, R., G. MAASS, and W. OEHLERT: Experimental infections of monkeys. Primates Med. 3, 138—139 (1969).

HAVEMANN, K., and H. A. SCHMIDT: Haematological findings in Marburg virus disease: evidence for involvement of the immunological system. In: Marburg Virus Disease, pp. 34—40. Springer-Verlag, Berlin-Heidelberg-New York, 1971.

HENDERSON, B. E., R. E. KISSLING, M. C. WILLIAMS, G. W. KAFUKO, and M. MARTIN: Epidemiological studies in Uganda relating to the "Marburg" agent. In: Marburg Virus Disease, pp. 166—176. Springer-Verlag, Berlin-Heidelberg-New York, 1971.

HENNESSEN, W.: Epidemiology of Marburg virus disease. Lab. Anim. 4, 137—142 (1969).

HENNESSEN, W.: Epidemiology of "Marburg virus" disease. In: Marburg Virus Disease, pp. 161—165. Springer-Verlag, Berlin-Heidelberg-New York, 1971.

HENNESSEN, W., O. BONIN und R. MAULER: Zur Epidemiologie der Erkrankung von Menschen durch Affen. Dtsch. med. Wschr. 93, 582—589 (1968).

HOFMANN, H., und CH. KUNZ: Das Verhalten des sogenannten „Marburg-Virus" in einigen Gewebekulturen. Zbl. Bakt. I. Abt. Orig. 208, 344—347 (1968).

HOFMANN, H., und CH. KUNZ: Komplementbindende Antikörper nach Infektion mit dem „Marburg-Virus" (Rhabdovirus simiae) beim Menschen. Zbl. Bakt. I. Abt. Orig. 209, 288—293 (1969 a).

HOFMANN, H., und CH. KUNZ: Interferonbildung im Gehirn weißer Säuglingsmäuse nach Infektion mit einigen Rhabdoviren. Zbl. Bakt. I. Abt. Orig. 211, 5—9 (1969 b).

HOFMANN, H., und CH. KUNZ: Ein mauspathogener Stamm des „Marburg-Virus"
(Rhabdovirus simiae). Arch. ges. Virusforsch. 32, 244—248 (1970).

HOFMANN, H., and CH. KUNZ: Cultivation of the Marburg virus (Rhabdovirus simiae)
in cell cultures. In: Marburg Virus Disease, pp. 112—116. Springer-Verlag, Berlin-
Heidelberg-New York, 1971.

HOFMANN, H., CH. KUNZ, H. ASPÖCK und A. RADDA: Zur Ökologie des sogenannten
„Marburg-Virus" (Rhabdovirus simiae). Zbl. Bakt. I. Abt. Orig. 212, 168—173
(1969).

HÜLSER, D.: Elektronenmikroskopische Untersuchungen an dem Erreger der Infektionskrankheit, die durch grüne Meerkatzen auf den Menschen übertragbar ist.
Zbl. Bakt. I. Abt. Ref. 215, 544—545 (1969).

HUMMELER, K., H. KOPROWSKI, and T. J. WIKTOR: Structure and development of
rabies virus in tissue culture. J. Virol. 1, 152—170 (1967).

JACOB, H.: The neuropathology of the Marburg disease in man. In: Marburg Virus
Disease, pp. 54—61. Springer-Verlag, Berlin-Heidelberg-New York, 1971.

JACOB, H., und H. SOLCHER: Über eine durch grüne Meerkatzen (Cercopithecus aethiops)
übertragene, zu Gliaknötchenencephalitis führende Infektionskrankheit („Marburger Krankheit"). Acta neuropath. (Berl.) 11, 29—44 (1968).

KAFUKO, G. W., B. E. HENDERSON, M. C. WILLIAMS, and R. E. KISSLING: Investigations in Uganda relating to the Marburg agent. In: Infections and Immuno-
suppression in Subhuman Primates (H. BALNER, and W. I. B. BEVERIDGE, eds.),
p. 45. Munksgaard, Copenhagen, 1970.

KALTER, S. S.: A serological survey of primate sera for antibody to the Marburg virus.
In: Marburg Virus Disease, pp. 177—187. Springer-Verlag, Berlin-Heidelberg-New
York, 1971.

KALTER, S. S., J. J. RATNER, and R. L. HEBERLING: Antibodies in primates to the
Marburg virus. Proc. Soc. exp. Biol. (N. Y.) 130, 10—12 (1969).

KAPLAN, M.: Collection and shipment of vervet monkeys. Primates Med. 3, 140—145
(1969).

KISSLING, R. E. (1968): see KALTER et al. (1969).

KISSLING, R. E., F. A. MURPHY, and B. E. HENDERSON: Marburg virus. Ann. N. Y.
Acad. Sci. 174, 932—945 (1970).

KISSLING, R. E., R. Q. ROBINSON, F. A. MURPHY, and S. G. WHITFIELD: Agent of
disease contracted from green monkeys. Science 160, 888—890 (1968).

KORB, G., H. BECHTELSHEIMER und P. GEDIGK: Die wichtigsten histologischen Befunde bei der „Marburg-Virus"-Krankheit. Dtsch. Ärztebl. 65, 1089—1096 (1968).

KORB, G., H. BECHTELSHEIMER und P. GEDIGK: Die Morphologie der Leber bei
der „Marburg-Virus"-Krankheit. In: Modern Gastroenterology, pp. 1307—1308.
F. K. Schattauer Verlag, Stuttgart-New York, 1969.

KORB, G., and W. SLENCZKA: Histologic findings in livers and spleens of guinea pigs
after infection by the Marburg virus. In: Marburg Virus Disease, pp. 123—124.
Springer-Verlag, Berlin-Heidelberg-New York, 1971.

KORB, G., W. SLENCZKA, H. BECHTELSHEIMER und P. GEDIGK: Die „Marburg-Virus"-
Hepatitis im Tierexperiment. Virchows Arch. Abt. A Path. Anat. 353, 169—184 (1971).

KUNZ, CH., and H. HOFMANN: Some characteristics of the Marburg virus. In: Marburg
Virus Disease, pp. 109—111. Springer-Verlag, Berlin-Heidelberg-New York, 1971.

KUNZ, CH., H. HOFMANN und H. ASPÖCK: Die Vermehrung des „Marburg-Virus" in
Aedes aegypti. Zbl. Bakt. I. Abt. Orig. 208, 347—349 (1968 b).

KUNZ, CH., H. HOFMANN, W. KOVAC und L. STOCKINGER: Biologische und morpho-
logische Charakteristika des Virus des in Deutschland aufgetretenen „Hämorrha-
gischen Fiebers". Wien. klin. Wschr. 80, 161—162 (1968 a).

MAASS, G., R. HAAS, and W. OEHLERT: Experimental infections of monkeys with the
causative agent of the Frankfurt-Marburg syndrome. Lab. Anim. H. 4, 155—165
(1969 b).

MAASS, G., J. MÜLLER, N. SEEMAYER, and R. HAAS: Production of kidney tissue cultures from African green monkeys, experimentally infected with the causative
agent of Frankfurt-Marburg-syndrome. Amer. J. Epidem. 89, 681—690 (1969 a).

MALHERBE, H., and M. STRICKLAND-CHOLMLEY: Human disease from monkeys (Marburg virus). Lancet ii, 1434 (1968).

MALHERBE, H., and M. STRICKLAND-CHOLMLEY: Studies on the Marburg virus. In: Marburg Virus Disease, pp. 188—194. Springer-Verlag, Berlin-Heidelberg-New York, 1971.

MARTINI, G. A.: Marburg agent disease: in man. Trans. royal Soc. trop. Med. Hyg. 63, 295—302 (1969).

MARTINI, G. A.: Marburg virus disease. Clinical syndrome. In: Marburg Virus Disease, pp. 1—9. Springer-Verlag, Berlin-Heidelberg-New York, 1971.

MARTINI, G. A., H. G. KNAUFF, G. BALTZER, H. A. SCHMIDT und F. H. KREUTZ: Das klinische Bild der Marburg-Virus-Krankheit, genannt „Marburger Affenkrankheit". Dtsch. Ärztebl. 65, 1675—1680 (1968 b).

MARTINI, G. A., H. G. KNAUFF, H. A. SCHMIDT, G. MAYER und G. BALTZER: Über eine bisher unbekannte, von Affen eingeschleppte Infektionskrankheit: Marburg-Virus-Krankheit. Dtsch. med. Wschr. 93, 559—571 (1968 a), German Med. Monthly XIII, 457—470 (1968).

MARTINI, G. A., und H. A. SCHMIDT: Spermatogene Übertragung des „Virus Marburg" (Erreger der „Marburger Affenkrankheit"). Klin. Wschr. 46, 398—400 (1968).

MARTINI, G. A., und R. SIEGERT: Die Marburg-Virus-Krankheit. Innere Medizin in Praxis und Klinik. Georg Thieme Verlag, Stuttgart. (Im Druck.)

MAY, G., und K. HERZBERG: Vergleich eines Affenseuche-Erregers mit einem Virus der Vesicularstomatitis-Gruppe. Zbl. Bakt. I. Abt. Orig. 211, 133—143 (1969).

MAY, G., und H. KNOTHE: Bakteriologisch-virologische Untersuchungen über die in Frankfurt/M. aufgetretenen menschlichen Infektionen durch Meerkatzen. Dtsch. med. Wschr. 93, 620—622 (1968), German Med. Monthly XIII, 518—520 (1968).

MAY, G., H. KNOTHE, D. HÜLSER und K. HERZBERG: Elektronenmikroskopische Befunde bei einer Affenseuche (Cercopithecus aethiops). Zbl. Bakt. I. Abt. Orig. 207, 145—148 (1968).

MELNICK, J. L., and R. M. McCOMBS: Classification and nomenclature of animal viruses, 1966. Progr. med. Virol. 8, 400—409 (1966).

MÜLLER, G.: Elektronenmikroskopische Partikelzählung in der Virologie. I. Zentrifugierröhrchen zur direkten Sedimentation von Viren auf Netzträger. Arch. ges. Virusforsch. 27, 339—351 (1969).

MURPHY, F. A., D. I. H. SIMPSON, S. G. WHITFIELD, I. ZLOTNIK, and G. B. CARTER: Marburg virus infection in monkeys — ultrastructural studies. Lab. Invest. 24, 279—291 (1971).

NITTNER, K.-R.: Measures taken by the Public Health Officials during the "Marburg virus disease". In: Marburg Virus Disease, pp. 216—219. Springer-Verlag, Berlin-Heidelberg-New York, 1971.

OEHLERT, W.: The morphological picture in livers, spleens, and lymph nodes of monkeys and guinea pigs after infection with the "vervet agent". In: Marburg Virus Disease, pp. 144—156. Springer-Verlag, Berlin-Heidelberg-New York, 1971.

PETERS, D.: Struktur und Entwicklung von Viren. Verh. dtsch. Ges. inn. Med. 75, 540—552 (1969).

PETERS, D.: Struktur, Vermehrung und Klassifikation des Marburg-Virus. Z. Versuchstierk. 12, 267—268 (1970).

PETERS, D., und G. MÜLLER: Die elektronenmikroskopische Erkennung und Charakterisierung des Marburger Erregers. Dtsch. Ärztebl. 65, 1831—1834 (1968).

PETERS, D., and G. MÜLLER: The Marburg agent and structures associated with Leptospira. Lancet i, 923—925 (1969 a).

PETERS, D., und G. MÜLLER: Zur Morphologie und Entstehung des Marburg-Virus. Zbl. Bakt. I. Abt. Ref. 215, 545 (1969 b).

PETERS, D., G. MÜLLER, and W. SLENCZKA: Morphology, development, and classification of the Marburg virus. In: Marburg Virus Disease, pp. 68—83. Springer-Verlag, Berlin-Heidelberg-New York, 1971.

ROBIN, Y., P. BRÈS, and C. CAMAIN: Passage of Marburg virus in guinea pigs. In: Marburg Virus Disease, pp. 117—122. Springer-Verlag, Berlin-Heidelberg-New York, 1971.

SCHUMACHER, W.: Legislative measures concerning the importation of monkeys. In: Marburg Virus Disease, pp. 223—225. Springer-Verlag, Berlin-Heidelberg-New York, 1971.

SHU, H. L., R. SIEGERT und W. SLENCZKA: Zur Pathogenese und Epidemiologie der Marburg-Virus-Infektion. Dtsch. med. Wschr. **93**, 2163—2165 (1968), German Med. Monthly **XIV**, 7—10 (1969).

SIEGERT, R.: not published (1967).

SIEGERT, R.: Konsequenzen aus der Marburger Affenvirus-Katastrophe. Umschau **68**, 664 (1968).

SIEGERT, R.: Probleme der Virusdiagnostik, dargestellt am Beispiel des Marburg-Virus. Verh. dtsch. Ges. inn. Med. **75**, 565—572 (1969).

SIEGERT, R.: The Marburg virus (vervet monkey agent). Modern Trends in Medical Virology **2**, 204—240 (1970 a). Butterworths, London.

SIEGERT, R.: Diagnostik, Pathogenese und Epidemiologie des Marburg-Virus beim Menschen. Z. Versuchstierk. **12**, 266—267 (1970 b).

SIEGERT, R., and H. L. SHU: not published (1967/1968).

SIEGERT, R., H. L. SHU und W. SLENCZKA: Isolierung und Identifizierung des ,,Marburg-Virus". Dtsch. med. Wschr. **93**, 604—612 (1968 a), German Med. Monthly **XIII**, 514—518 (1968).

SIEGERT, R., H. L. SHU und W. SLENCZKA: Nachweis des Marburg-Virus beim Patienten. Dtsch.med.Wschr.**93**,616—619(1968b), German Med. Monthly **XIII**,521—524(1968).

SIEGERT, R., H. L. SHU und W. SLENCZKA: Zur Diagnostik und Pathogenese der Infektion mit Marburg-Virus. Dtsch. Ärztebl. **65**, 1827—1830 (1968 c).

SIEGERT, R., H. L. SHU, W. SLENCZKA, D. PETERS, and G. MÜLLER: Detection of the so-called green monkey agent. Proc. IV. Congreso Latinamericano de Microbiologia, Lima/Peru, 26 Nov.—2 Dec. (1967 a).

SIEGERT, R., H. L. SHU, W. SLENCZKA, D. PETERS und G. MÜLLER: Zur Ätiologie einer unbekannten, von Affen ausgegangenen menschlichen Infektionskrankheit. Dtsch. med. Wschr. **92**, 2341—2343 (1967 b), German Med. Monthly **XIII**, 1—3 (1968).

SIEGERT, R., and W. SLENCZKA: Laboratory diagnosis and pathogenesis. In: Marburg Virus Disease, pp. 157—160. Springer-Verlag, Berlin-Heidelberg-New York, 1971.

SIMPSON, D. I. H.: personal communication (1969 a).

SIMPSON, D. I. H.: Marburg agent disease: in monkeys. Trans. roy Soc. trop. Med. Hyg. **63**, 303—309 (1969 b).

SIMPSON, D. I. H.: Isolation of the causal agent. Primates Med. **3**, 135—137 (1969 c).

SIMPSON, D. I. H.: Marburg virus disease: experimental infection of monkeys. Lab. Anim. H. **4**, 149—154 (1969 d).

SIMPSON, D. I. H.: Vervet monkey disease, transmission to the hamster. Brit. J. exp. Path. **50**, 389—392 (1969 e).

SIMPSON, D. I. H.: Marburg virus: a review of laboratory studies. In: Infections and Immunsuppression in Subhuman Primates, (H. BALNER, and W. I. B. BEVERIDGE, eds.), pp. 39—44. Munksgaard, Copenhagen, 1970.

SIMPSON, D. I. H., E. T. W. BOWEN, and W. F. BRIGHT: Vervet monkey disease: experimental infection of monkeys with the causative agent, and antibody studies in wild-caught monkeys. Lab. Anim. **2**, 75—81 (1968 a).

SIMPSON, D. I. H., I. ZLOTNIK, and D. A. RUTTER: Vervet monkey disease, experimental infection of guinea-pigs and monkeys with the causative agent. Brit. J. exp. Path. **49**, 458—464 (1968 b).

SLENCZKA, W.: not published (1968).

SLENCZKA, W.: Growth of Marburg virus in Vero cells. Lab. Anim. H. **4**,143—147(1969a).

SLENCZKA, W.: Zum Verhalten des Marburg-Virus in Verozellen. Zbl. Bakt. I. Abt. Ref. **215**, 545—546 (1969 b).

SLENCZKA, W.: not published (1970).

SLENCZKA, W., H. L. SHU, G. PIEPENBURG und R. SIEGERT: Antigen-Nachweis des ,,Marburg-Virus" in den Organen infizierter Meerschweinchen durch Immunfluoreszenz. Dtsch. med. Wschr. **93**, 612—616 (1968), German Med. Monthly **XIII**, 524—529 (1968).

SLENCZKA, W., R. SIEGERT und G. WOLFF: Nachweis komplementbindender Anti-körper des Marburg-Virus bei 22 Patienten mit einem Zellkultur-Antigen. Arch. ges. Virusforsch. **31**, 71—80 (1970).

SLENCZKA, W., and G. WOLFF: Biological properties of the Marburg virus. In: Marburg Virus Disease, pp. 105—108. Springer-Verlag, Berlin-Heidelberg-New York, 1971.

SLENCZKA, W., G. WOLFF, and R. SIEGERT: A critical study of monkey sera for the presence of antibody against the Marburg virus. Amer. J. Epidem. **93**, 496—505 (1971).

SMITH, C. E. G.: Microbiological research at Porton. Vervet monkey disease. Nature (Lond.) **218**, 1114 (1968).

SMITH, C. E. G., D. I. H. SIMPSON, E. T. W. BOWEN, and I. ZLOTNIK: Fatal human disease from vervet monkeys. Lancet ii, 1119—1121 (1967).

SOLCHER, H.: Neuropathological findings in experimentally infected guinea pigs. In: Marburg Virus Disease, pp. 125—128. Springer-Verlag, Berlin-Heidelberg-New York, 1971.

Special Studies Laboratory, NCDC: Follow-up obscure disease related to African monkeys. Morbidity and Mortality Weekly Report **17**, 223 (1968).

STILLE, W., and E. BÖHLE: Clinical course and prognosis of Marburg virus ("green-monkey") disease. In: Marburg Virus Disease, pp. 10—18. Springer-Verlag, Berlin-Heidelberg-New York, 1971.

STILLE, W., E. BÖHLE, E. HELM, W. VAN REY und W. SIEDE: Über eine durch *Cercopithecus aethiops* übertragene Infektionskrankheit („Grüne-Meerkatzen-Krankheit", "Green Monkey Disease"). Dtsch. med. Wschr. **93**, 572—582 (1968), German Med. Monthly **XIII**, 470—478 (1968).

STOJKOVIĆ, LJ., M. BORDJOŠKI, A. GLIGIĆ, and Ž. STEFANOVIĆ: Two cases of cercopithecus-monkeys-associated haemorrhagic fever (some data on etiology, epidemiology and epizootiology). In: Marburg Virus Disease, pp. 24—33. Springer-Verlag, Berlin-Heidelberg-New York, 1971.

STOJKOVIĆ, LJ., A. GLIGIĆ, M. BORDJOŠKI, and Ž. STEFANOVIĆ: Some data on etiology, epidemiology, and epizootiology of Cercopithecus-associated hemorrhagic fever. Report: 8 Int. Congr. trop· Med. Malar., Teheran, 7—15 Sept. 1968.

STRICKLAND-CHOLMLEY, M., and H. MALHERBE: Marburg virus. Lancet ii, 476 (1970).

STRICKLAND-CHOLMLEY, M., and H. MALHERBE: Examination of South African primates for the presence of Marburg virus. In: Marburg Virus Disease, pp. 195—202. Springer-Verlag, Berlin-Heidelberg-New York, 1971.

TODOROVITCH, K., M. MOCITCH, and R. KLAŠNJA: Clinical picture of two patients infected by the Marburg vervet virus. In: Marburg Virus Disease, pp. 19—23. Springer-Verlag, Berlin-Heidelberg-New York, 1971.

WATERSON, A. P.: Measles virus. Arch. ges. Virusforsch. **16**, 57—80 (1965).

WILLIAMS, M. C., B. E. HENDERSON, P. M. TUKEI, J. M. ELLICE, M. LULE, and Y. SSENKUBUGE: Haemorrhagic disease in West German laboratory workers. E. Afr. Virus Res. Inst., Ann. Rep. No. 17, 43—45 (1968), Government Printer, Entebbe/Uganda.

ZLOTNIK, I.: Marburg agent disease: pathology. Trans. roy Soc. trop. Med. Hyg. **63**, 310—323 (1969).

ZLOTNIK, I.: "Marburg disease." The pathology of experimentally infected hamsters. In: Marburg Virus Disease, pp. 129—135. Springer-Verlag, Berlin-Heidelberg-New York, 1971.

ZLOTNIK, I., and D. I. H. SIMPSON: Culture of vervet-monkey-disease agent. Lancet ii, 458 (1968).

ZLOTNIK, I., and D. I. H. SIMPSON: The pathology of experimental vervet monkey disease in hamsters. Brit. J. exp. Path. **50**, 393—399 (1969).

ZLOTNIK, I., D. I. H. SIMPSON, W. F. BRIGHT, E. T. W. BOWEN, and DEE BOTTER-HATTON: Growth of vervet monkey disease agent in BHK cell cultures. Brit. J. exp. Path. **49**, 311—314 (1968 a).

ZLOTNIK, I., D. I. H. SIMPSON, and D. M. R. HOWARD: Structure of the vervet-monkey-disease agent. Lancet ii, 26—28 (1968 b).

ZWILLENBERG, L. O., M. H. JENSEN, and H. L. ZWILLENBERG: Electron microscopy of the virus of viral haemorrhagic septicaemia of rainbow trout (Egtved virus). Arch. ges. Virusforsch. **17**, 1—19 (1965).

VIROLOGY MONOGRAPHS
DIE VIRUSFORSCHUNG IN EINZELDARSTELLUNGEN